NATIONAL INSTITUTE FOR SOCIAL WORK TRAINING SERIES

NO. 19

HELPING THE AGED
A FIELD EXPERIMENT IN SOCIAL WORK

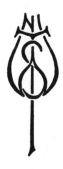

Publications by the
National Institute for Social Work Training
Mary Ward House, London W.C.1

NO. 1 SOCIAL WORK AND SOCIAL CHANGE
by Eileen Younghusband

NO. 2 INTRODUCTION TO A SOCIAL WORKER
produced by the National Institute for Social Work Training

NO. 3 SOCIAL POLICY AND ADMINISTRATION
by D. V. Donnison, Valerie Chapman and others

NO. 4 SOCIAL WORK WITH FAMILIES
Readings in Social Work, Volume 1
compiled by Eileen Younghusband

NO. 5 PROFESSIONAL EDUCATION FOR SOCIAL WORK IN BRITAIN
by Marjorie J. Smith

NO. 6 NEW DEVELOPMENTS IN CASEWORK
Readings in Social Work, Volume 2
compiled by Eileen Younghusband

NO. 7 THE FIELD TRAINING OF SOCIAL WORKERS
by S. Clement Brown and E. R. Gloyne

NO. 8 DECISION IN CHILD CARE
A Study of Prediction in Fostering Children
by R. A. Parker

NO. 9 ADOPTION POLICY AND PRACTICE
by Iris Goodacre

NO. 10 SUPERVISION IN SOCIAL WORK
by Dorothy E. Pettes

NO. 11 CARING FOR PEOPLE
The 'Williams' Report
on the Staffing of Residential Homes

NO. 12 SOCIAL WORK AND SOCIAL VALUES
Readings in Social Work, Volume 3
compiled by Eileen Younghusband

NO. 14 EDUCATION FOR SOCIAL WORK
Readings in Social Work, Volume 4
compiled by Eileen Younghusband

NO. 15 CHILD CARE: NEEDS AND NUMBERS
by Jean Packman

NO. 16 THE VOLUNTARY WORKER IN THE SOCIAL SERVICES
Chairman of Committee: Geraldine M. Aves

NO. 17 A PLACE LIKE HOME: A PIONEER HOSTEL FOR BOYS
by David Wills

NO. 18 THE ADOPTION OF NON-WHITE CHILDREN
by Lois Raynor

NO. 19 HELPING THE AGED
by E. Matilda Goldberg with others

NO. 20 VOLUNTEERS IN PRISON AFTER-CARE
by Hugh Barr

NO. 21 HOMELESS NEAR A THOUSAND HOMES
by Bryan Glastonbury

NO. 22 HUMAN DEVELOPMENT
by Eric Rayner

NO. 23 PLANS AND PROVISIONS FOR THE MENTALLY
HANDICAPPED
by Margaret Bone, Bernie Spain and F. M. Martin

HELPING THE AGED

A FIELD EXPERIMENT IN SOCIAL WORK

by

E. MATILDA GOLDBERG

with
ANN MORTIMER
BRIAN T. WILLIAMS

with a Foreword by
RICHARD M. TITMUSS

London
GEORGE ALLEN & UNWIN LTD
RUSKIN HOUSE   MUSEUM STREET

FIRST PUBLISHED IN 1970

Second impression 1972

© *George Allen & Unwin Ltd 1970*

ISBN 0 04 362019 1 CASED

ISBN 0 04 362020 5 PAPER

PRINTED IN GREAT BRITAIN BY
REDWOOD PRESS LIMITED
TROWBRIDGE, WILTSHIRE

RESEARCH TEAM

E. Matilda Goldberg, A.A.P.S.W. Director of Research
Mary B. Speak, B.SC., PH.D Statistician
Phyllis E. Baldock, B.A., A.I.M.S.A. Social Work Assessor
Ann Mortimer, B.A. Social Work Assessor
Brian T. Williams, M.B., B.S., D.P.H., D.P.M. Medical Assessor
Edith K. M. Harrison, A.A.P.S.W. Social Worker
Michael G. Picardie, B.A., A.A.P.S.W. Social Worker
Anne Vickery, A.A.P.S.W. Social Work Interviewer
Elizabeth A. Howe, Statistical Assistant
Mair Wynn Griffiths, Administrative Secretary

Computer Analysis by Whittle Data Services

ADVISORY COMMITTEE

CONTENTS

———

9

ACKNOWLEDGEMENTS

Many people besides the research team have contributed to this study and to the completion of the book.

First, we want to acknowledge the generous grant by the Department of Health and Social Security, which had the foresight to support a hazardous and unpredictable study. We are grateful to them for making the study possible and for the encouragement they have given throughout.

We wish also to pay tribute to the wholehearted co-operation received from all the staff of the welfare department of the local authority concerned. This co-operation was expressed in the allocation of excellent premises and facilities, in the warm acceptance of all members of the research team as colleagues, and in the conscientious adherence to the administrative procedures necessary to ensure the smooth and efficient working of the experiment. Above all, this collaboration was shown in the welcome extended to an experiment which involved close scrutiny of some of the department's own work. The success of this complex combined operation augurs well for experiments in other social work organizations in this country.

We want to thank the medical officer of health of the local authority and the general practitioners who readily co-operated with our medical assessor.

The consultative committee gave us valuable advice and support throughout and individual members were ready to be consulted freely between committee meetings.

We could not have attempted the diet study without the expert advice and guidance of Miss Jean Marr, dietitian of the Social Medicine Research Unit of the Medical Research Council, who devoted time and knowledge to the study.

We wish to thank Professor Henry Meyer of the School of Social Work of the University of Michigan. While he was a Fulbright Scholar at this Institute he acted as consultant to the study and we benefited from his unique experience in the field of social work research.

We also want to acknowledge the help of our colleague Miss June Neill who analysed the 'consumer' data at very short notice.

Dr Austin Heady read the final drafts as an independent expert; his comments and suggestions were of great value.

Professor Richard Titmuss, in spite of the heavy demands continually made on him, kindly agreed to write a Foreword and in doing this made valuable comments about the manuscript. We deeply appreciate his help.

Above all we wish to thank Mr Robin Huws Jones, Principal of the Institute, whose support and encouragement were forthcoming throughout this venture and whose detailed comments on every aspect of the drafts contributed immeasurably to the book's coherence and readability.

Last but not least we thank our secretary, Mrs Jarmaine Haddon, not only for retyping drafts with cheerful efficiency but for being ever alert to errors and inconsistencies, assuming responsibilities far beyond her secretarial work.

Finally we acknowledge our debt to the old people themselves, many of whom were very aged and frail and who patiently answered questions the social and medical assessors put to them before and after the experiment. Without their faithful co-operation the study could not have been carried out at all. We hope that what we have learnt from them will eventually benefit other old people who need the help of the social services.

FOREWORD
by RICHARD M. TITMUSS

General practitioners, medical officers of health, psychiatrists, health visitors, school teachers, social workers and others with personal service duties in the health and welfare fields have all been criticized in recent years for their failure as organized professional groups to assess their effectiveness in the actual performance of their respective service roles and functions. Even the corridors of universities have been torn with academic dissension when confronted with the challenge, presented by the Prices and Incomes Board in 1970, of determining criteria for the assessment of a 'good teacher'.

In part, the debate is about the exercise of power by these professions and the values underlying its use in situations of social control. In part, it reflects the growth of consumer reaction groups and rising demands for consultation and participation. And in part, it has been generated by critics of specific education and training systems; critics who ask, for example, for evidence justifying the professional training of social workers. This search for ways and means of measuring professional performance in terms of consumer opinion is to some extent connected with the fact that economists, increasingly preoccupied with cost-benefit analysis, are beginning to question whether more investment in education and the allocation of more resources for health care can be objectively justified on economic criteria. Higher education, in particular, cannot apparently be shown to 'pay'.

These general and specific issues of professional effectiveness and the exercise of power are not peculiar to Britain. They are being raised in all industrialized societies with highly-developed systems of health and welfare. Nor is the questioning being confined to the assessment of the professional role. It is being recognized that the worker cannot be abstracted from the structure of resources and facilities – the universe of 'service instrumentalities'. We cannot ask 'how effective is social work' without also asking questions about the performance of the institutions and services within and around which the worker operates.

Similarly, we cannot inquire about quality standards of family doctoring without taking account of all the facilities and tools, medical and social, which are or might be at the service of the practitioner and the patient's family. What then – we are thus led to ask – are the objectives of these institutions and services and how do those who staff them perceive their ends and means? What, in the absence of criteria of profitability, is 'success' for a hospital out-patient department, a group practice, a social work agency, an area office of the Supplementary Benefits Commission, and how is it or might it be measured?

To get people 'off the books', to close files, to record 'not seen again' or 'referred to X', to discharge from clinic, hospital and other institution and to get some adults into work and others into wedlock are all indicators of something – and certainly measures of institutional productivity and professional desk clearance – but they tell us little about the effective performance of the service role from the perspective of the patient, client, student or consumer. All professional élites lay claim to 'busyness' and the more 'busyness' they themselves generate and then record somewhere as items of service may justify, in trade union terms, higher salaries or status promotions. Such output activities do not in themselves, however, validate professional training, nor are they necessarily indices of effective treatment, particularly when consumer needs are multiple, many-sided and involve more than one institution, agency or service.

It is relatively easy, of course, for academic social scientists to criticise the 'helping' professions; many of the critics find satisfaction and certainty in self-defined entrepreneurial success goals. Industrious denigration can often spell academic promotion. But for members of the 'helping' professions the goals are often ambiguous, conflicting or unclear. Where they are apparent and acceptable to both the professional worker and the client they almost always relate to elements in physical functioning; the doctor, for instance, who chooses correctly – or by chance – the right antibiotic and can record recovery, or the probation officer who arranges for a client's facial disfigurement to be removed thus enabling him to compete successfully in the labour market.

But for the great majority of people seen by social workers it is hard to determine mutually acceptable criteria of success or failure. What is 'improvement' or 'deterioration', for whom in the family, on what time-scale and on whose assessment? In formulating such questions we have to remember that in most cases the mechanistic test of work, often applied on Calvinistic principles by members of some professions, is not applicable; we cannot so easily dispose of as successes or failures society's 'outcasts' or 'inadequates' and those who are not and may never be susceptible to positive criteria of 'regular work.'

Another difficulty in evaluating social work activities lies in the fact that 'effectiveness' heavily depends not only on the general infrastructure of social service institutions but on their variety, distribution, accessibility and range of specialized functions; from particularly experienced home helps for motherless families to half-way homes for young male schizophrenics discharged from mental hospitals. If these are absent, inaccessible or grossly inadequate the social worker is as much handicapped as the doctor is today in most parts of Africa. The worker may thus be forced into or restricted to 'therapeutic counselling', just as the general practitioner in Edwardian England was restricted to little but a stethoscope or as American social workers are today in the virtual absence of personal social services in many disadvantaged areas.

There cannot be one unambiguous goal for social work; human needs and desires are complex, interdependent, simultaneously rational and irrational, and often in conflict. Nor is there one unambiguous objective for the social services. It would be terrifying if there were and if we thought there could be. All one is left with (or all I am left with) is the philosopher's thought that increasing sensitiveness to the claims of others (and claims which cannot be wholly satisfied on the material criteria of the market) is one important element in the definition of moral progress in society.

To use the word in a quite different sense, Miss Goldberg and her colleagues have deployed sensitivity in their attempt in this study to assess the effectiveness of social work with elderly clients of a local authority welfare department. The results will be keenly debated, closely dissected and criticized with regard to the formulation of their hypotheses, the validity of the assessment techniques employed and the interpretation of the results. They deserve to be and for four substantial reasons.

For one thing, this study represents the first controlled field experiment in Britain in the complex and diffuse area of activities which we call social work. All those who participated are to be commended not only for their respective contributions but for the high ethical standards which were observed and maintained throughout the duration of the experiment.

Second, because old age was chosen as the area of need within which to assess the effectiveness of trained social workers in 'promoting welfare'. In Chapter 11 Miss Goldberg discusses the advantages and disadvantages of this choice, methodological and interpretative. I would have said, had I been asked when the experiment was being designed, that the disadvantages would outweigh the advantages. 'Improvement' among the elderly – particularly the demanding, the lonely and the apathetic elderly – cannot be spectacular over a relatively short period of time; deterioration can. Now after reading the report I am not so sure. One critical element justifying social work and justifying training is the listening role – an element often overlooked or misinterpreted by the critics of the profession. Listening not to oneself but to what others may be trying to say is an essential part of social diagnosis as well as medical diagnosis. From it flows (in D. H. Lawrence's words) 'sympathetic consciousness'. It has also a value in itself, social, cultural and moral, in implying and expressing respect for the dignity of others in a world which values speed, busyness, efficiency and activity. The dominance of these values should lead us to ask: who is listening in society for the sounds and symptoms of need for help? How do we within local administrative structures institutionalize the listening role and in ways which signal to those concerned that the message has been received?

These questions are critical because the perception and articulation of need flows from disciplined listening; such purposive listening is an essential prerequisite to effective action. 'Effective', in this context, means practical action attuned to client priorities, combined simultaneously with psychological help. For a range of unexpressed and unmet needs – from money to the re-establishment of relationships with relatives – to be sensitively identified some groups more than others require more social work skills in listening. This study demonstrates that one such group are the elderly. The demonstration lies in the evidence presented that listening led to skilled action; action that was practical and, according to the independent assessors, effective. It further suggests that those who were trained listened as effectively to those whose needs were greatest. Thus, there was relatively more action on their behalf; more resources were mobilized. In other words, the trained workers functioned selectively; they concentrated more practical aid and more psychological effort on those who appeared to need help most. This finding, sharply at variance from the general run of utilization studies, could not, however, have emerged without the relatively generous infrastructure of services in the area studied. With fewer universal resources and facilities available selectivity becomes less possible.

The third reason for commending this study lies in the methodological challenge it presented and the ways in which attempts were made to resolve the formidable conceptual and technical problems referred to earlier in this note. It seems to the writer that whatever qualifications may be attached to some of the findings what cannot be disputed is that methodologically this study is more advanced than similar social work experiments in the United States and other countries.

Lastly, it has to be said that the experiment involved as a research project lengthy and complex teamwork arrangements between the social work agencies concerned, statutory and voluntary, and the research team. Miss Goldberg is to be congratulated for successfully organizing these arrangements and for thus making, in this report, a major contribution to the advancement of knowledge about social work and its future in the development of social policy in Britain.

PREFACE

In 1965 a team including social workers, a physician and a statistician embarked on a study which attempted to assess the effectiveness of social work with elderly clients of a local authority welfare department. The aims of the study were:

1. To assess the social and medical condition and needs of a defined sample of old people aged 70 and over who applied to a welfare department because they were in need of domiciliary services, social support or residential accommodation.

2. To compare the services received from statutory or voluntary agencies with the help that appeared to be necessary in view of the social and medical condition of the old persons.

3. To assess how the use of trained and experienced social workers can contribute to the welfare of the old person and his or her family.

The report is divided into four parts.

Part I begins with a discussion of some theoretical and practical issues which affect the objectives of social work and any assessment of its effectiveness.

The following chapter considers the advantages and disadvantages of choosing the problems of the aged for a field experiment in social work. It describes the pilot phase of the study in which hypotheses were clarified and assessment techniques developed.

Part II is concerned with the first two aims of the study. It gives an objective picture of the social circumstances and medical conditions of the 300 welfare clients who were assigned to the experiment; it then explores what help these old people were already receiving from their families, friends and neighbours and from the social services, and tries to assess what additional help was necessary for a reasonably comfortable existence.

Part III deals with the social work experiment. The social and medical characteristics of the randomly assigned 'special' (experimental) and 'comparison' (control) groups are compared and found to be essentially similar. We then give a comparative account of the social work which in the special group was undertaken by trained social caseworkers and in the comparison group by the authority's welfare officers who though often experienced and trained 'on the job' had not received full-time training in social work. We proceed to assess the outcome of social work in the two groups by measuring and comparing changes in the clients' material conditions, their physical and social functioning and their subjective attitudes. This is followed by a description of the consumers' opinions about their contacts with the social workers and the help they had received from them.

Finally, in Part IV tentative conclusions are drawn and their implications considered for social work among the aged, for the organization of services and for the training of social workers.

PART I

Objectives and Methods

I

THE OBJECTIVES OF SOCIAL WORK – CAN THEY BE DEFINED AND ASSESSED?

In our affluent welfare state social workers are in great demand and their numbers are steadily increasing as expectations of improved social conditions and better physical and mental health continue to rise. The Seebohm Report (H.M.S.O. 1968) pointed to many gaps and deficiencies in the personal social services and argued forcibly for an extension of social work services and their greater unity and autonomy. Increasing resources are devoted to the training of social workers. Social workers are progressing towards a professional entity with the founding of the British Association of Social Workers. Social work has arrived.

At the same time there has been a swelling chorus of voices asking: What is social work? What do social workers do and how effective are they?

Among the first determined voices to be heard was Barbara Wootton's, some ten years ago (Wootton 1959). She observed that 'in a very few years practically the whole profession has succeeded in exchanging the garments of charity for a uniform borrowed from the practitioners of psychological medicine'. She suggested that the modern social worker (like her Victorian predecessor) was confusing economic difficulties with personal failure and misconduct and that undue attention to the casework process and the casework relationship was deflecting attention away from problems created by evil environments. Since the modern social worker saw her concern to be with psychological maladjustment rather than material need, she found it harder to say what she was driving at.

More recently, with the rediscovery of poverty as a primary evil and a respectable complaint worthy of attention in its own right, doubts about the methods employed by social workers and especially by caseworkers, about the objectives they pursue and the effectiveness of their efforts, have become more insistent on both sides of the Atlantic.

In America social workers have been accused of deploying their resources where they are least needed, of neglecting the poor and the severely disordered, 'putting commitment to a method before human needs', methods, moreover, which have not been shown to be effective (Scott Briar 1968). Like Wootton, Scott Briar takes social workers to task for retreating from an array of functions as 'social brokers, advocates, reformers and participants in social policy' to the one exclusive function as therapists, adopting a 'psychiatric disease' model, as their frame of reference. He argues that casework methods are based on explanatory theories which do not provide knowledge of how to change conditions.

Meyer and his colleagues, in their famous field experiment in social work with adolescent girls, have criticized the almost exclusive concentration of the caseworkers dealing with these girls on self-understanding and on attitudes (Meyer et al. 1965). They suggest that social work might achieve better results if it was directed towards helping clients to change their situations and their goals.

In Great Britain, Sinfield (1969) in a recent Fabian pamphlet also deplores the narrow interpretation of the modern social worker's role and the profession's tendency to look inward into its own processes which, in his view, leads to neglect of the client's views and of the goals to be achieved. He thinks that social workers fail to validate techniques because they often assume that they are checking their own work in the process of casework itself. The criteria for success therefore, Sinfield argues, are the social workers' own and not their clients'. This view is confirmed, to a limited extent, by studies of medical social workers, who expressed dissatisfaction with their efforts as they were not able to use their casework skills to the full (Moon 1965, Butrym 1968). However, the clients in Butrym's study expressed considerable satisfaction about the support and practical help they had received from the medical social workers.

The suggestions that social workers apply their skills most successfully to those who need them least and that the psycho-therapeutic model of social work based mainly on the exploration of the client–worker relationship may not be appropriate in certain types of case, are reinforced by a recent study of probationers (Davies 1969). Probationers who had good relationships with their parents and a supportive environment were likely to make a good relationship with their probation officer and to avoid further court appearances, while those whose environments were disturbed and who had very poor relationships with their parents also made a poor contact with their probation officers and were likely to get into trouble again. In other words, the probation officers were most successful with those who needed them least and failed with those who needed help most.

The validity of certain other cherished notions, for instance the superiority of long-term casework, has recently been challenged by Reid and Shyne's wholly unexpected findings, that families receiving help limited to eight interviews made more progress than similar families who had long-term treatment (Reid and Shyne 1969). Furthermore the strong suggestion emerges from this and other investigations (Mayer and Timms 1969) that clients prefer active and goal-directed help to passive exploratory techniques which aim at explanation and understanding, rather than specific change.

A serious handicap in evaluating social work is the vagueness of the descriptions of what social workers actually do. Social workers are apt to write in somewhat pompous and complex language about the transactions between themselves and their clients, emphasizing the vagaries, complexities and subtleties of the casework process. They have been relatively silent about the vast amount of down to earth practical help and advice they also afford their clients, as if ashamed of this side of social work, though there are some notable exceptions (Sheppard 1966, Parkinson 1970). Nor has much been said about the social worker's functions of linking clients with a host of voluntary and statutory agencies in the community and of interpreting their needs to these agencies. Hence descriptions of social work activities are often somewhat partial and misleading and many people believe that the majority of caseworkers are immersed in long-term intensive casework dealing with their clients' intra-psychic and unconscious conflicts, discussing and interpreting childhood experiences, and so on.

The few careful studies that have been carried out suggest that the reality is very different and more oriented towards the present inter-action between the client and his surroundings and more concerned with practical help than these notions would suggest. Some of these studies show that only around 1 per cent to 2 per cent of the case-workers' responses in interviews with clients who were experiencing difficulties in family relationships dealt with intra-psychic causes of behaviour or the childhood origins of current difficulties (Reid 1967, Hollis 1968, Mullen 1968).

All these findings indicate that the time is ripe for critically examining the goals and methods of social work and in particular those of social casework. At the same time one cannot ignore the formidable difficulties which stand in the way of a truly scientific evaluation of so-called 'effectiveness' in this field of human endeavour.

Social workers have traditionally been landed with, or sought out the 'outcasts' in society, and those whose handicaps are long-standing or irreversible: those who do not respond to active medical treatment or cannot make use of the social services provided. Social workers are concerned with the disabled, the subnormals, the so-called 'character disorders', the deprived and the disadvantaged. It is true that social workers have also become increasingly concerned with so called preventive functions – for example in child guidance and marriage guidance. However, in these spheres too they are often dealing with severely disturbed families, and the original idea of giving guidance to families at the earliest signs of disturbance in order to prevent serious trouble later, has long since been lost sight of.

How, then, can we determine criteria of success in such an ill-defined field of social failure and disabilities of all kinds? There are no tests to show, as in some fields of medicine, whether the invading bacilli have been eradicated or the cancerous cells stopped from multiplying. One may even be at a loss how to interpret apparent improvement; intervention may merely cause the underlying pathology of a behavioural disorder to choose a different path and it may presently erupt in a different form. Or 'improvement' may set up a chain reaction which will throw out of balance a long-established social equilibrium. For instance, when a submissive and chronically unemployed husband starts work and becomes more self-reliant as a result of social work help, this may upset the equilibrium of his marriage: his dominating wife, who is used to a dependent husband and holding the reins herself, may become depressed, feel useless and lose her customary self-confidence in the face of her husband's new, more assertive and masculine role.

Another difficulty in defining criteria of success and failure is that theories of social work intervention are based on different sociological and psychological theories of human functioning (Plowman 1969). For instance behaviour therapists base their treatment largely on learn-

ing theories. Faulty functioning is perceived as learnt behaviour which
has to be unlearnt and redirected towards healthier goals without the
necessity of understanding why these maladaptations have arisen. For
behaviour therapists, outward behaviour rather than inner experience
constitutes the criterion of success or failure. The psycho-dynamic
school of psychology to which most social workers subscribe is not
nearly so concerned with specific goals. The psycho-dynamically
oriented social worker will aim at increasing the client's understanding
of the experiences which have caused his problems and at the client's
recognition of his own contribution to these problems. Such 'insight'
may lead to a change in behaviour and attitude, or it may enable the
client to feel better about himself and the world around him and to live
more comfortably with his difficulties, whether they are within himself
or part of his environment. But as a psycho-analyst has recently said
with remarkable frankness: 'it still remains uncertain as to how far
insight either relieves stress or modifies behaviour' (Storr 1966).

There is thirdly the existentialist position of 'being in the world',
which is a unique experience not susceptible to final analysis. What is
often ignored in our society and in the helping professions – so the
argument runs – is the role of the other significant person who may
define a situation as a problem situation to serve his own needs and
thus actually create or exacerbate something which may have started as
a simple oddity or as a variant of an ordinary situation (Laing 1968).
What in our society is labelled mental illness or deviance is intelligible
as a reaction to social forces surrounding the 'sick' individual – a
family, a social or political system which drive him into madness. The
so-called 'cures' may deprive the deviant of his human dignity and his
ability to protest or to opt out. It is the social structure of society and
its dominant values which need adjusting rather than the individuals,
who are the victims of an irrational social situation. The healers, the
'labellers' may be as sick or more sick than those they are attempting to
cure and community action and shared social experience are seen as
more appropriate.

Fourthly, the socialist or social reform position (already touched on
in Wootton's and Sinfield's criticisms of social work) has implications
for the aims of social work and hence for criteria of success and failure.
If the problem is one of scarce or maldistributed human and economic
resources and of unmet material needs then – the social reformers
postulate – the social workers should aim at changing policy, ensuring

that the client gets his rights and their concern should be with community services, rather than with personal change and adaptation.

Both the third and fourth positions may underestimate the role of individual pathology in creating and aggravating social and psychological problems; but whatever position we adopt the relative influences of family, social and unique experiential factors are woven together in a way which makes it difficult to arrive at a clear theoretical standpoint and unambiguous social work aims.

It seems then that social work like other helping professions is concerned with a wide variety of social and psychological conditions whose aetiology is often only partially understood and which may not be susceptible to 'cure'. The appropriateness and efficacy of casework methods are open to question, the possible goals of social work raise a whole host of problems of the individual in society, since they 'concern the manifold problems of the human condition and the difficulties we all have in living' (Storr, op. cit.).

However, as we shall show presently, there are a number of more limited goals capable of definition and assessment which social workers can and do pursue in their attempts to help their clients.

For instance, in a case of chronic disability increased physical and social activity or resumption of work may be valid goals; in a family with an anxious and disturbed child who makes no progress at school an improvement in the mother/child relationship, accompanied by a decrease in the child's disturbance and better marks at school may be relevant criteria of success. In dealing with old people a modest improvement in their morale and a higher degree of safety and comfort resulting from increased domiciliary services may constitute measurable objectives.

Assuming that we are able to define some goals which permit the formulation of criteria of success and failure in relation to specific problems, and that we can describe the 'treatment' given in different cases, how can we be sure that the outcome – favourable or unfavourable – is due to the social work carried out, rather than to the myriad of events in the lives of our clients which have nothing to do with social work?

One answer is by subjecting two essentially similar, randomly chosen groups of clients to two different kinds of social work. We could then postulate that the intervening events will affect both groups in a similar fashion and that the only consistently varied experience will be the type of social work received. Any differences that emerged between the groups at the end of such an experiment could then be reasonably attributed to the different types of social work rather than to the other random influences they may have experienced in the intervening period (Suchman 1967).

In order to carry out such a controlled experiment it is essential to observe five conditions:

1. We need two samples of clients which are as similar as possible and at the same time representative of the kind of population we wish to study. This equivalence is usually achieved by randomly assigning the chosen population to an 'experimental' and a 'control' group.

2. The treatment to be tested will have to be administered to the experimental group and a recognizably different treatment to the control or comparison group. In this way the *relative effectiveness of different treatments* will be put to the test.

3. We need to specify the treatments which are being evaluated.

4. It is essential to spell out what is meant by a 'successful' result, e.g. what the criteria of success are we wish to measure.

5. These criteria will have to be measured in both groups in as unbiased a fashion as possible *before* and *after* treatment; that is to say the assessors carrying out these measurements should be unaware of who is in the experimental and the control groups and be independent and separate from the social workers engaged in treatment.

The results of six field experiments in social work, all of them carried out in the USA, are now available. The first was carried out by the Community Service Society of New York in the late fifties and early sixties. A defined population aged 60 and over were randomly assigned to three alternative services: the usual service provided by the Society's district offices, a short-term service limited to four interviews in which the applicant was assigned either to a caseworker or a public health nurse, whoever seemed more appropriate, and a collaborative service in which the caseworker and the public health nurse collaborated in giving as intensive and long-term help as was necessary (Blenkner et al. 1964).

The second experimental study was undertaken in the late fifties in New York City on a group of 200 adolescent girls with certain social and psychological problems; 100 of these girls received skilled social casework help at a youth consultation centre and the other half no specific treatment (Meyer *et al.*, op. cit.). The third experiment was carried out in Chemung County in New York in the early sixties among 100 multi-problem families, half of whom received intensive social casework and half the services of public assistance officers (Brown 1968). The fourth study took place at the Benjamin Rose Institute, Cleveland, Ohio, and was concerned with a sample of 150 people over the age of 60 living in the community who were judged to be mentally incapable of caring adequately for themselves: half received skilled casework services, combined with maximum use of community resources and the other half had whatever services happened to be available to them in the community (Blenkner *et al.* 1967). In the fifth experiment, personal, neighbourhood and community resources were made available to tenants aged 60 and over in four public housing projects in New York by mature in-service-trained workers under the supervision of a trained social worker. In order to assess the effectiveness of the service the emotional, social and physical functioning of the elderly populations in the four serviced housing projects were compared with two similar populations in housing projects not receiving these services (Community Service Society 1969).

The sixth investigation aimed at assessing the relative effectiveness of different patterns of casework service – planned short-term service and open ended long-term service – in alleviating family problems (Reid and Shyne, op. cit.).

The results of these experiments were somewhat disappointing. They showed very small, if any gains in outcome among the experimental groups which had received skilled casework or other forms of special social help; and the experiment in which short- and long-term casework was compared, as already mentioned, produced the surprising result that short-term help appeared to be more effective than long-term treatment among families with similar and often severe disturbances in family relationships. However, this finding was entirely consistent with the Community Service Society's earlier study on ageing (Blenkner *et al.* 1964, op. cit.) in which the long-term service was found to be inferior to short-term service on most indices used.

Certain criticisms have been voiced about some of these experiments: the motivation of clients who had been randomly assigned to forms of treatment they had not sought was questioned; the vaguely defined objectives of the social work effort and the relevance of the treatment methods used have been critically discussed; it has also been suggested that the effects of social work help may be visible only after a much longer time interval than was possible to allow for in these studies; and finally doubt has been cast on the validity of the criteria chosen to indicate success or failure (MacDonald 1966, Perlman 1968).

We hope that the design and methods used in the field experiment to be reported in the following pages meet some of these criticisms, and we shall return to them in our concluding discussion.

References

Blenkner, M., Jahn J., and Wasser, E. (1964): *Serving the Ageing: An experiment in social work and public health nursing*, Community Service Society of New York, Institute of Welfare Research (mimeographed).

Blenkner, M., Wasser, E. and Bloom, M. (1967): *Protective Services for Older People*, Progress Report for 1966–67, Community Service Society of New York, Institute of Welfare Research (mimeographed).

Brown, Gordon E. (1968): *The Multi-Problem Dilemma: A social research demonstration with multi-problem families*, Scarecrow Press Inc.

Butrym, Zofia (1968): *Medical Social Work in Action*, Occasional Papers on Social Administration, No. 26, Bell.

Community Service Society of New York (1969): *Senior Advisory Service for Public Housing Tenants* (mimeographed).

Davies, Martin (1969): *Probationers in their Social Environment*, H.M.S.O.

H.M.S.O. (1968): *G.B. Report of the Committee on Local Authority and Allied Persons Social Services*, Cmnd. 3703.

Hollis, Florence (1968): 'A Profile of Early Interviews in Marital Counselling', *Social Casework*, Vol. 49, No. 1.

Laing, Ronald D. (1968): *Intervention in Social Situations*, Association of Family Caseworkers.

Macdonald, Mary E. (1966): 'Reunion at Vocational High: An Analysis of Girls at Vocational High: An Experiment in Social Work Intervention', *Social Service Review*, XL, No. 2.

Mayer, John E. and Timms, Noel (1969): 'Clash in Perspective between Worker and Client', *Social Casework*, Vol. 50, No. 1.

Meyer, H. J., Borgatta, E. F. and Jones, W. C. (1965): *Girls at Vocational High: An experiment in social work intervention*, Russell Sage Foundation.

Moon, Marjorie (1965): *The First Two Years*, Institute of Medical Social Workers.

Mullen, Edward J. (1968): 'Casework Communication', *Social Casework*, Vol. 49, No. 9.

Parkinson, Geoffrey (1970): 'I Give Them Money', *New Society*, 5th February.

Perlman, Helen H. (1968): 'Casework and the Case of Chemung County', in: *The Multi-Problem Dilemma*, op. cit.

Plowman, D. E. G. (1969): 'What are the Outcomes of Casework?' *Social Work*, Vol. 26, No. 1.

Reid, William J. (1967): 'Characteristics of Casework Intervention', *Welfare in Review*, Vol. 5, No. 8.

Reid, W. J. and Shyne, Ann W. (1969): *Brief and Extended Casework*, N.Y. Columbia University Press.

Scott, Briar (1968): 'The Casework Predicament', *Social Work*, Vol. 13, No. 1.

Sheppard, M. L. (1966): 'The Social Worker's Use of Material and Practical Aid'; *The British Journal of Psychiatric Social Work*, Vol. 8, No. 3.

Sinfield, Adrian (1969): 'Which Way for Social Work?', *Fabian Tract 393*, Fabian Society.

Storr, A. (1966): 'The Concept of Cure', in: Rycroft, C. (editor): *Psychoanalysis Observed*, Constable.

Suchman, Edward A. (1967): *Evaluative Research*, New York. Russell Sage Foundation.

Wootton, Barbara (1959): *Social Science and Social Pathology*, Allen and Unwin.

2

THE DEVELOPMENT OF ASSESSMENT TECHNIQUES AND THE FORMULATION OF HYPOTHESES

When our study was designed and begun in 1965 none of the results of the American social work experiments were available, except those of the Community Service Society's project *Serving the Ageing* (Blenkner *et al.* 1964, op. cit.). One of us had returned to a social work setting – the National Institute for Social Work Training – after a long period in social medicine research in which clinical trials of different treatments based on random assignment of patients to experimental and control groups were common currency. It therefore seemed quite natural to venture into a clinical trial designed to test the effectiveness of social work in a particular sphere.

As mentioned in the introduction we chose the field of old age and our aims were three-fold: to ascertain the social and medical condition and needs of a sample of old people aged 70 and over newly referred to a local authority welfare department; to compare services received with services needed; and to assess how effective trained social workers were in promoting the welfare of these aged persons.

There were three strong reasons for choosing the field of old age for such a study:

1. The increasing challenge that community care of the elderly presents to social workers.

2. The unique opportunity which the staffing conditions in this field offered at the time for a controlled experiment in which the relative effectiveness of work carried out by professionally trained and untrained social workers could be tested.

3. The possibilities which social work with the aged presents to quantify social work effort because much of the help required is of a practical kind.

There were also some obvious disadvantages which are related to the small changes one could reasonably expect in this age group.

The Increasing Challenge. Readers will be familiar with the great increase in numbers, both absolute and proportionate of old people in this century. The number of those over 75, when disability tends to become chronic and serious, has grown fourfold for men and fivefold for women. At the same time their own children have not increased proportionately because of the sharp decrease in the birth rate since Victorian times. In addition many of the married and single daughters who could care for their aged parents during the day are likely to be employed outside their homes.

A number of important pioneer studies carried out over the last twenty years in this and other countries[1] have clearly outlined the general conditions of the aged in our society, where the most serious problems lie, and what gaps remain in social and medical provisions and services. The most important source of information in this country is the national survey of a random sample of about 4,000 persons over the age of 65 carried out by Townsend and his colleagues as part of a cross-national study (Townsend and Wedderburn 1965, Shanas *et al.* 1968). We now know that only about $4\frac{1}{2}$ per cent of the elderly live in institutions including hospitals, that around 12 per cent receive domiciliary health and welfare services and that the family, far from misusing welfare services still dwarfs the social services in caring for their elderly relatives, particularly in illness and infirmity. It has also become apparent that the elderly are an economically disadvantaged group, that their housing conditions are often highly unsuitable to their needs and that substantially more old people need services than are receiving them. This applies to almost all the available services, but particularly to home helps, meal services, chiropody, hearing aids, sheltered housing and residential accommodation. A case for major social action in relation to income and housing and for a very considerable expansion of domiciliary services has been established. What, in addition can social work most usefully contribute to the well-being of the growing number of aged citizens and how can one ensure that scarce resources of trained manpower are used most effectively?

A Unique Opportunity. In 1965–66 when the study began most welfare

[1] See starred references at end of this chapter.

departments employed welfare officers who had not yet been able to take a professional training in social work. This situation offered an opportunity for testing experimentally what contributions trained social workers could make to the welfare of elderly clients, by comparing the outcomes of their work with the results achieved by their experienced but professionally unqualified colleagues. This meant that a test of the relative effectiveness of two treatments could be devised without depriving anyone of the customary welfare services, as would have happened in a controlled experiment in which social work intervention was compared with no intervention. Ideally, from a scientific point of view, the design of an experiment to test the effectiveness of social work would have been to locate a random sample of old people in a defined area, to assess their functioning and needs and then to randomly assign one-third of those found in need of help to trained social workers (the 'experimental' group), another third to the customary welfare services (the 'contrast' group) and to leave one-third as they were (the 'control' group). After a specified period one would have reassessed the sample and compared the different treatments with one another and with the untreated group. Such a study would have been ethically unacceptable to the researchers as it would have meant leaving some old people, known to be in need, without help.

A field experiment within the setting of a welfare department was not merely the only feasible one; it was also the most economic way, as it eliminated the necessity of screening large numbers of households and old people to find those 'in need'. By definition most elderly applicants to a local authority welfare department are 'in need'. More important, however, such an experiment was the most relevant test. Since no one would argue that old people in need should not be helped at all, the real question is *what kind of help*. By comparing the outcomes of different 'treatments' one might gradually arrive at the most appropriate type of assistance. For instance one could possibly indicate those aspects in the care of the elderly in which skilled professional social work appears to be essential to achieve worthwhile results and those areas in which a less highly trained or different kind of help could be at least as effective. However, such a design implied that the differences in outcome could never be spectacular, since both the experimental and the 'comparison' group were likely to receive a substantial amount of help.

The Measurement of Social Work Input. A third advantage in choosing the field of old age was that we were dealing with a group which had many practical needs calling for concrete help and delivery of services and close liaison with a variety of other social and medical agencies. These kinds of activity can be described and measured fairly satisfactorily and we were thus able to quantify and compare social work effort in the two groups.

Possible Disadvantages of Choosing Elderly Clients. It may be said that social work with the aged in the setting of a welfare department is an unpromising field and not a fair test for the effectiveness of social work. Such critics may rightly point out that one could not expect much change or improvement among the very old. This is true in some respects. No one would hope to influence or to change basic attitudes and styles of life in old age. Yet it can be a very promising field if one interprets the term 'social work' with the breadth it deserves. It will then include concern with the external social situation, with the acceptable delivery of appropriate services, with the enrichment of social relationships in the community as well as with the therapeutic impact of the casework relationship on feelings of depression, frustration and loneliness. Also, old age and disability come to all, if they live long enough. Since there is less reluctance than formerly to use the welfare department, especially in an area in which a good deal of publicity is given to the services available, the group with which we are concerned may well be a more normal cross-section responding to help in less complex ways than obviously pathological groups such as problem families, or mentally ill patients and their families.

Length of Intervention and Motivation. Since help had to be offered and to produce results in this world rather than the next, a comparatively short period of social work – between nine months and a year – seemed to be the only realistic and feasible one. This again fitted in well with the requirements of an experiment which cannot be extended over an indefinite period.

The problem of motivation was not likely to intrude as much as it might have done in some other experimental studies of random samples of potential clients who had not sought treatment, for example the adolescent girls at a Vocational High School in New York who were offered help at a Youth Consultation Centre more or less out of the blue (Meyer *et al.*, op. cit.). All the participants in our study had applied or had been referred for help to the local authority welfare department.

In retrospect, the field of the aged turned out to be a good one to choose for an experimental study, both from the point of view of the urgency of the problems presented to the welfare services and of fulfilling the conditions necessary to carry out a field experiment that was scientifically sound, and relevant to the questions which needed exploring as well as ethically acceptable.

The Development of Assessment Techniques
An extensive pilot study exploring both social and medical aspects in which around 100 old people were seen, and lasting about a year, was carried out in the welfare department of an outer London borough. The aims of the pilot study were manifold: to develop measures for assessing the social and medical conditions and physical functioning of old people aged 70 and over referred to a welfare department, to find out whether such independent assessments could be carried out under the umbrella of a welfare department, and whether very old people were able to co-operate in a fact-finding kind of social and medical inquiry. We also tried to estimate the losses through death, hospitalization, etc., over 9 to 10 months of social work and the amount of co-operation likely to be forthcoming in a second social and medical interview after a period of several months. Finally we sought to formulate hypotheses about the kind of changes that skilled social work might bring about in the conditions of old people.

It soon became clear both in the social and medical part of the pilot study, that provided the interviews did not take more than about an hour and a half almost all the old welfare clients were able to co-operate; indeed many expressed pleasure about the interest shown in their welfare. A somewhat smaller proportion – around 90 per cent – consented to a health assessment. It was also reassuring to find that old people over the age of 80 who constituted half of the pilot 'sample', were able to answer questions as lucidly as those under 80.

Since the aim of the study was to compare many variables at two points in time it was necessary to develop highly structured questionnaires. One of the main problems was to obtain sufficient information on which to base a social and medical assessment and reasonably accurate measurements of change, without overburdening this rather infirm group of very old people. The range of information sought had therefore to be limited, so as to allow the interviews to be completed in about one to one and a quarter hours.

In order to achieve comparability with other social and medical studies of the elderly, we tried to use wherever possible measures which had already been tested, for example Townsend's personal incapacity and household incapacity measures (Townsend and Wedderburn, op. cit.), questions relating to the amount of contact with family, friends and neighbours, and certain questions concerned with loneliness and social attitudes. Some of these questions had to be simplified somewhat to fit in with the impaired memories of these clients whose average age was very much higher than that of most other samples studied. The development of measures of the old people's 'morale' and general attitudes proved difficult, yet it was an area in which we thought that changes might well occur following social work intervention. Several questions were eventually formulated related to loneliness, satisfaction and dissatisfaction in various spheres of living, as well as a series of statements about the old people's attitudes to the world around them with which they could agree or disagree. (It will be shown later that some of the answers to these attitude questions were highly correlated and formed a cluster emerging as a 'factor' in the component analysis and proving a sensitive measure of change.)

Most of the areas we tapped in order to assess the old people's medical and social conditions and any changes resulting from social work had been explored before in other medical and social surveys. We added one new aspect to a socio-medical experiment of this kind, namely the old people's diet. We were anxious to detect those old people who clearly had an inadequate diet and to discover whether social workers, by devoting some attention to those with poor diets were able to bring about any improvement as part of their social work effort. Under the guidance of a consultant dietitian, Miss Jean Marr, of the M.R.C. Social Medicine Unit, we finally decided to concentrate our efforts on the old person's main sources of protein, since we could only devote a small part of the interview to the dietary inquiry. Questions were formulated about the source and content of the main meal, about the quantity of milk, eggs, cheese and bread bought weekly, and about the numbers of helpings of fish or meat eaten other than at the main meal. On the basis of the answers to these questions a scoring system was developed which enabled us to divide the old people into groups, a top group, a middle group and a bottom group in relation to protein intake. As a test of its validity the scoring system developed for this study was applied to the diets of 60 elderly women not part of the present study living alone in London (Exton Smith *et al.* 1965). These women, all aged 70 and over, had recorded and weighed their diets and thus a comparison could be made between actual weights and the scores. A good agreement was obtained between the two methods in placing these women into top, middle and bottom thirds and thus some confidence can be placed in the diet measures employed in this study, especially since the main aim was to detect merely the bottom third, those who almost certainly had an inadequate diet. In the main study we informed the social workers in both the experimental and the comparison groups of welfare clients whose diet scores fell into the bottom group.

In order to test the reliability of the observations recorded in the interview schedules, Miss Goldberg (the director of the study) and Mrs Mortimer (the social work assessor) paid ten joint visits towards the end of the pilot phase. Interviews were conducted in turn while both completed the questionnaires which were subsequently compared. Few discrepancies occurred in relation to factual questions but rather more on the assessments which were based on subjective judgements. Most of these differences were due to lack of precise criteria rather than to a difference of opinion about the actual situation. From the ensuing discussions more precise criteria emerged on which judgements were to be based and which were used as a guide when we took on a second social work assessor. Comparison of the distribution of ratings based on subjective judgements between the two assessors in the main study showed them to be strikingly similar.

The structured social interview which finally emerged lasted on average an hour and a quarter; it explored the old people's physical environment, their financial situation, their mobility and ability to perform the most basic personal and household tasks, what help they were receiving and what additional services they thought they needed. Questions were asked about their diet, their activities in and outside their home, their contacts with children, other relatives and neighbours and the help they received from them. Finally, an attempt was made to explore the applicants' attitudes to their health, their present situation and to life in general and how they saw the world around them.[1]

Immediately after the interview the social work assessor (using

[1] Copies of the social questionnaire can be inspected in the Institute's library.

previously defined criteria) rated the state of the old persons' housing and amenities and made a subjective assessment of their contentment. The assessor also recorded what she considered the applicant needed in the way of additional help and services. Lastly, she noted her impression of the old persons' main problems, how great she felt the need for social work intervention was and how much change she expected from this.

In the medical part of the pilot study we took cognizance of the evidence that the refusal rates are usually higher in medical studies of the aged in which full clinical examinations are proposed – around 20 per cent – than in those where an interview only, or an interview with a partial clinical examination is attempted – between 2 per cent and 4 per cent.[1] We therefore decided early on to combine an interview with a partial clinical examination.

In nearly all the recorded surveys of the elderly the help of general practitioners has been enlisted in approaching old people, or in supplying supplementary clinical information. The general practitioners of the old people in the pilot study were approached by the medical investigator to ensure that they had no objection to a health assessment; no objections were made. Several methods of obtaining supplementary information from the general practitioners were tested for their relative effectiveness: approach in person, by telephone and by post. Eventually a short postal inquiry proved to be effective; and since it was also the most economic method it was adopted in the main study.

When attempting to categorize the medical states of old people, Hobson & Pemberton (op. cit.) remarked upon the inadequacy of a medical diagnosis for describing the extent of disability in an old person. Chronic bronchitis for example might render one person breathless on the slightest exertion, while another, though having a cough, producing phlegm, might experience no breathlessness. Yet some knowledge of the conditions from which the old people suffered was essential in order to formulate an opinion of the prognosis, irrespective of treatment. For instance, a rapidly progressive medical condition could nullify the social worker's efforts to help an old person overcome the effects of a disability; on the other hand by arranging medical care the social workers might indirectly ameliorate the condition and improve the outlook by the time the second medical assessment

[1] See references: Sheldon 1948; Hobson & Pemberton 1955; Parsons 1962; Williamson et al. 1964; Kay et al. 1964.

was made. The medical assessor arrived at a tentative diagnosis on the basis of the old person's reported symptomatology, the physical signs which he observed without the client undressing and any signs of psychiatric illness which appeared during the course of the interview; the results of the analysis of a blood sample taken at the end of the interview were also available. Supplementary information was obtained from the old person's general practitioner about the diagnosis of any condition present and any current treatment. From these data the medical assessor was able to construct a fairly complete picture of the diagnosis and probable prognosis of the old person's medical condition. Whenever the medical investigator discovered a condition which needed prompt treatment he passed the information to the old person's general practitioner.

Standardized procedures for detecting disease prevalent in older people such as ischaemic heart pain, intermittent claudication (Rose 1962) and hypothyroidism (Wayne 1960) did not prove suitable tools for assessing this very aged group. Most of the Medical Research Council's questionnaire on respiratory symptoms (Fairbairn et al. 1959) also proved to be inappropriate except a group of four questions relating to breathlessness which were easily understood. The answers enabled us to grade the reported breathlessness according to severity and to compare the extent of this disabling symptom before and after the period of social work.

Serious confusion related to organic brain syndrome can be socially very disrupting and it was therefore important to assess the extent of the confusion present. The Tooting Bec Hospital questionnaire (Doust et al. 1953) is a validated instrument which discriminates between confused and lucid patients in a psychiatric hospital population. It was possible to adapt this questionnaire to the needs of these old people living outside hospital and to validate it with another population living in the community (Williams, in press).

Depression is widely experienced by old people living at home.[1] Moreover, it is a symptom which might be alleviated by social work. A series of six questions was constructed which probed the old person's tendency to feel depressed. The extent to which the old person felt depressed was measured by marking and rating on graphic linear scales the responses made to the six questions. These six questions have

[1] See references: Tunstall 1966; Parsons 1962, Kay et al., Williamson et al., op. cit.

been validated by showing that they discriminated clearly between a group of people being admitted to a psychiatric hospital diagnosed as suffering from affective disorder; a group entering old people's homes; and a group attending a Derby and Joan club (see Williams, in press).

Disabilities arising from impaired mobility, sight and hearing seriously affect the quality and enjoyment of an old person's life. Objective assessments of these disabilities were developed in order to measure the effects of any medical care, aids or adaptations arranged by social workers.

The various aspects of the medical assessment which had been developed piecemeal throughout the pilot stage were finally assembled into a schedule.[1] The structured interview and partial clinical examination used in the main study lasted on average one hour.

The development of these social and medical instruments served two purposes; to describe the social and medical conditions of the sample of old people who were to be the subjects of the experiment and to provide criteria on which changes could be measured.

Measuring Changes

In considering possible changes that might result from social work we anticipated that they might occur in four different areas.

1. *Environmental changes* could occur in relation to housing, or housing amenities, with regard to income and the provision of services.

2. *Changes in functioning* could take place as a result of social work or medical help. Such changes might be detectable in functional movement, in personal and household capacity, in the state of health both in relation to minor disabilities and major disease, in dietary habits, in general activities and interests and in the type and extent of social contacts.

3. *Changes in subjective attitudes* might be registered in the feelings the old people express, for example the amount of depression and loneliness experienced, satisfactions with various aspects of living and attitudes towards the world around them.

4. *The assessors may detect changes* in the extent and nature of the old people's needs, the type and severity of problems experienced and in the general contentment conveyed in the interview.

[1] Copies of the medical questionnaire can be inspected in the Institute's library.

In short, the criteria chosen ranged from objectively observable and verifiable facts to subjective attitudes and feelings expressed by the clients themselves. The criteria also included clinical judgements made by the social-work assessors and the medical investigator in relation to disability, the nature and extent of the old people's needs for additional social work help and more global clinical judgements about their general state of health and the degree and type of social problems experienced.

Initially it was also intended to assess and measure the burden on the family, but this proved to be beyond the resources of the study.

Hypotheses to be Tested. In accordance with these wide ranging criteria the following hypotheses were formulated.

General Hypotheses
As a result of social work:

1. More clients in the special group will survive to the time of the second assessment than in the comparison group.
2. More clients in the special group will show positive changes in their social and medical condition than in the comparison group.
3. Fewer clients in the special group will be admitted to institutional care than in the comparison group.

Specific Hypotheses
As a result of social work:

1. Fewer clients in the special group will show deterioration in scores for self care and household capacity than in the comparison group.
2. There will be no difference between the special and comparison group in relation to improved amenities, e.g. means of heating, toilet arrangements, cooking facilities, adaptations and aids.
3. More clients in the special than in the comparison group will improve their social contacts with family, neighbours and friends.
4. More people in the special than in the comparison group will develop interests and activities, e.g. clubs, workgroups, holidays, home library, church contacts, hobbies.
5. More clients in the special than in the comparison group will show improvement in their attitudes to their present situation as measured by the attitude score.

6. At the end of the social work period clients in the special group will have fewer social needs than clients in the comparison group and the decrease in needs will be greater in the special than in the comparison group.

7. Clients who were initially severely emotionally disturbed or had seriously disturbed interpersonal relationships will show greater improvement in the special than in the comparison group.

References

Adams, G. F. and Cheeseman, E. A. (1951): *Old People in Northern Ireland*, Northern Ireland Hospitals Authority, Belfast.

Bamlett, R. and Milligan, H. C. (1963): Health and Welfare Services, and the over 75s: 'A Geriatric Survey at West Hartlepool', *Medical Officer*, 109, pp. 379–85.

* Brockington, F. and Lempert, S. M. (1966): *The Social Needs of the Over-80s*, Manchester University Press.

* Cole, D. with Utting, J. (1962): *The Economic Circumstances of Old People*, Occasional Papers on Social Administration, No. 4, Codicote Press.

Doust, J. W., Schneider, R. A., Talland, G. A., Walsh, M. A. and Barker, G. B. (1953): The Correlation between Intelligence and Annoxemia in Senile Dementia, *Journal of Nervous and Mental Diseases*, 117, pp. 383–98.

Edge, J. R. and Nelson, I. D. M. (1963): Survey of Arrangements for the Elderly in Barrow in Furness, *Medical Care*, I, pp. 202–18.

Exton-Smith, A. N. and Stanton, B. R. (1965): *Report of an Investigation into the Dietary of Elderly Women Living Alone*, King Edward's Hospital Fund for London, 34 King Street, London, E.C.2.

Fairbairn, A. S., Wood, C. H. and Fletcher, C. M. (1959): Variability in Answers to a Questionnaire on Respiratory Symptoms, *British Journal of Preventive and Social Medicine*, 13, pp. 175–93.

Greenlees, A. and Adams, J. (1950): *Old People in Sheffield*, Sheffield Council of Social Service.

* Harris, A. and Woolf, M. (1962): *Health and Welfare of Older People in Lewisham*, Government Social Survey, H.M.S.O. London.

* Harris, A. with Clausen, R. (1968): *Social Welfare for the Elderly*, H.M.S.O. London.

Household Food Consumption and Expenditure, 1966: Annual Report of the National Food Survey Committee (1968), H.M.S.O. London.

* Hobson, W. and Pemberton, J. (1955): *The Health of the Elderly at Home*, Butterworth.

Kay, D. W. K., Beamish, P. and Roth, M. (1964): Old Age Mental Disorders in Newcastle-Upon-Tyne, *British Journal of Psychiatry*, Vol. 110, pp. 146–59.

Kilpatrick, G. S. and Hardisty, R. M. (1961): 'The Prevalence of Anaemia in the Community', *British Medical Journal*, I, pp. 778–82.

* Parsons, P. L. (1962): *The Health of Swansea's Old Folk*, unpublished M.D. Thesis, University of Wales.

* Parsons, P. L. (1965): 'Mental Health of Swansea's Old Folk', *British Journal of Preventive and Social Medicine*, 19, pp. 43–47.

Report on Services for the Elderly in the Metropolitan Borough of Lewisham (1964): A Committee sponsored by the King Edward's Hospital Fund for London, 34 King Street, London, E.C.2.

* Richardson, I. M. (1964): *Age and Need*, E. & S. Livingstone, Edinburgh.

Rose, G. A. (1962): *The Diagnosis of Ischaemic Heart Pain and Intermittent Claudication in Field Surveys*, Bulletin of the World Health Organization, 27, pp. 645–58.

* Shanas, E., Townsend, P., Wedderburn, D., Friis, H., Milhoj, P. and Stehouwer, J. (1968): *Old People in Three Industrial Societies*, Routledge, London.

* Sheldon, J. H. (1948): *The Social Medicine of Old Age*, Oxford University Press.

* Townsend, P. (1957): *The Family Life of Old People*, Routledge, London.

* Townsend, P. (1962): *The Last Refuge*, Routledge, London.

* Townsend, P. and Wedderburn, D. (1965): *The Aged in the Welfare State*, Occasional Papers on Social Administration, No. 14, Bell.

* Tunstall, J. (1966): *Old and Alone*, Routledge, London.

Wayne, E. J. (1960): Clinical and Metabolic Studies in Thyroid Disease, *British Medical Journal*, I, pp. 78–90.

* Williamson, J., Stokoe, I. H., Gray, S., Fisher, M., Smith, A., McGhee, A. and Stephenson, E. (1964): 'Old People at Home. Their Unreported Needs', *Lancet* I, pp. 1117–20.

Williams, B. W. (in press): *The Use of the Modified Tooting Bec Questionnaire to Measure Cognitive Function in a Community Survey of the Elderly*.

Williams, B. W. (in press): *An Instrument to Measure some Aspects of Depression in the Elderly*.

PART II

The Baseline of the Experiment

3

THREE HUNDRED AGED WELFARE CLIENTS THEIR SOCIAL AND MEDICAL CONDITIONS AND THEIR NEEDS

The Area

The field experiment took place in a London borough south of the river. This area was chosen mainly because it contained the average national proportion of people over 65, namely 12 per cent; it was a fairly typical inner London working-class borough with better than average social provision for the elderly, both in relation to the services provided and to the proportion of social workers employed per head of population; and lastly both the council members and the staff of the welfare department were enthusiastic about co-operating in such an experiment.

The population of the borough in 1966 was about 300,000, and the number of old people aged 70 and over was about 22,000 (7 per cent of the borough population). The northern part of the borough is densely populated and partly given over to wharves, factories and offices; the south is more suburban and middle class in character. The population like that of all inner London boroughs is declining. Many families are moving to the outer suburbs and commute into the borough for work. The area contains a wide variety of housing. Wartime bombing and subsequent redevelopment of large areas are causing the break-up of old neighbourhoods, although there are still some streets of two-storey terraced houses and others of three- or four-storey terraces in multi-occupation. In addition, there are old tenement blocks with inadequate amenities as well as an ever-increasing number of modern council flats.

The welfare department is well known in the neighbourhood and goes out of its way to bring its services to the notice of the public and invite people in need to apply for help. The area is comparatively well served by settlements, day centres and clubs. The spirit of neighbourliness is still very much alive in parts of the borough despite the redevelopment and the consequent uprooting of large sections of the community.

The Sample
Since our main aim was to evaluate the impact of social work on a group of elderly people in need we decided:

1. to accept only *newly* referred cases:
2. to restrict the study to those aged 70 and over when losses through death, frailty and disability mount and make independent existence in the community increasingly difficult;
3. to include all applicants in need of social work help, except any who were unlikely to remain in the community.

This meant that all new cases over 70 who were placed on one of the department's registers (blind, physically handicapped or 'elderly at risk') were eligible excepting emergencies which were likely to be admitted to residential homes or hospitals within a month of referral and those clients whose need appeared to be slight (such as a holiday only or a minor aid). Our target was to assess the social and medical condition of 300 old people. This allowed for a probable loss of a third during the course of the experiment ensuring that around 200 applicants would remain in the study until its conclusion. In order to achieve this we had to contact 330 suitable cases (Table III. 1). The reasons for excluding 30 are given in the table.

TABLE III. I

THE SAMPLE

Number of referred cases meeting criteria included in the study 300
Number of referred cases meeting criteria not included in the study 30

Died prior to assessment	8
Part III prior to assessment	4
In hospital for more than one month	6
Too ill/dying	1
Already having visits from Welfare Department	5
Wife already has Welfare Department visits	1
Moved, present address not known	1
First visit revealed very minor problems only	4
	30

The final sample consisted of 79 men and 221 women (for details see Table III. 4); just under half (46 per cent) were over the age of 80.

Sources and Reasons for Referral to the Welfare Department. 35 per cent of the old people were referred by health agencies, that is to say, hospitals, the local authority health department (largely through their home help service) or general practitioners (Table III. 2). 31 per cent

TABLE III. 2

SOURCES OF REFERRAL OF 300 OLD PEOPLE TO WELFARE DEPT.

Sources	Number of people	%
Hospitals	47	16
Health Dept. (inc. home help)	34	11
G.P.	23	8
Relatives	42	14
Self	26	9
Friends/neighbours	24	8
Dept's welfare officers and councillors	45	15
Statutory and voluntary agencies	44	15
Miscellaneous	13	4
Not known	2	1
Total	300	101

had come to the notice of the department because either the old person or relatives or friends and neighbours made a request for domiciliary services and other kinds of practical help. The department's welfare officers themselves picked up a number of cases on their rounds or through their meals-on-wheels reviews.

Most of the requests were either directly or indirectly for domiciliary services and for amenities such as aids, adaptations, clubs and holidays (Table III. 3). Only 8 per cent of all the applications raised the question of residential accommodation explicitly. Other applications were phrased in terms of the problems the applicants experienced such as illness, loneliness, difficulty in managing. Thus both the sources of referral and the nature of the requests suggest that the applicants' main needs were for domiciliary help and supporting services in order to enable them to carry on an independent existence in their own homes.

TABLE III. 3

MAIN REASONS FOR REFERRAL TO WELFARE DEPARTMENT

Reasons	Number of people	%
Domiciliary services requested, including aids and adaptations	70	23
Physical handicap including poor sight	52	17
Illness of client's relative	48	16
Other services (e.g. clubs, holidays)	33	11
Residential care	24	8
After-care on discharge from hospital	20	7
Housing	20	7
Isolation, loneliness, inter-personal difficulties	17	6
Finance	7	2
Miscellaneous	9	3
Total	300	100

Method of Approach and Response by Clients. During a period of 10 months every newly referred person over the age of 70 was notified to the research team on a specially designed form, after a preliminary visit by one of the department's welfare officers.

During this first visit the applicant's immediate problems were explored and any necessary emergency action taken. If the old person met the criteria for inclusion in the study he or she was visited by one of the social work assessors.

Although nearly half the old people were over 80 and almost a third had disabilities impeding the interview such as deafness, confusion, discomfort or illness, it was possible to complete the lengthy questionnaire for 290 applicants – 97 per cent; a shortened version was used for 9 others and 1 very disturbed old lady (the only case of classic schizophrenia in the sample) refused to be interviewed at all. Two hundred and seventy or 90 per cent 'co-operated well' in the interview, readily giving full information. This very high completion rate and degree of co-operation are clearly related to the social work assessors' credentials. They came from the welfare department to which the applicants had turned for help. One also needs to remember that these old folk had plenty of leisure to talk in some detail about their daily lives, their children, friends and neighbours. At the end of the visit the social work assessor asked for permission for the medical assessor to call. Most of the old people agreed and the medical assessor was able to see 283 of them (94 per cent).

With the exception of a few old ladies who mistrusted the young doctor – and one in particular who thought he might be a thug and his Harpenden skinfold calipers a revolver – they were pleased to receive such a thorough medical examination from the 'welfare doctor'.

The Old People

If we compare the age, sex and marital state of this sample of welfare applicants with persons in a similar age group in their area we find that there were proportionately more people over eighty and fewer men; fewer of them were married and more widowed and divorced (Table III. 4 and Table III. 5). This underrepresentation of males is probably associated with women living longer; hence men are less likely to be left alone and to need welfare services. The prevalence of the widowed and divorced in our sample is reflected in the fact that nearly two-thirds (64 per cent) lived alone compared with 25 per cent of old people in a similar age group in a national study (Townsend and Wedderburn, op. cit.). This picture ties in with the finding that widowed, divorced and

TABLE III. 4

AGE

Welfare clients compared with borough population*
(Percentage distributions)

Age	Men		Women	
	Welfare clients	Borough population*	Welfare clients	Borough population*
(yrs)	(N=79)	(N=7,731)	(N=221)	(N=15,825)
70–74	32	45	19	41
75–79	30	32	33	32
80–84	20	16	26	18
85–89	13	6	17	7
90	5	1	5	2
Totals	100	100	100	100

Source: *1961 Census County Report for Greater London* (Table 2).

*The 1966 Sample Census does not break down age into groups above 75 years, but comparing where possible the 1961 Census, the 1966 Sample Census does not show any real differences

single old people make greater demands on the hospital services than those living in families (Abel-Smith and Titmuss 1956). It is worth noting that the widowed and divorced, rather than the single are over-represented in our group: possibly people who have been single all their lives have learnt to be self-sufficient, even in old age and infirmity though other selective factors may have been at work.

TABLE III. 5

MARITAL STATE
Welfare clients compared with borough population
(Percentage distributions)

Marital state	Men		Women		Total	
	Welfare clients (N=79)	Borough population (N=6,950)	Welfare clients (N=221)	Borough population (N=15,060)	Welfare clients (N=300)	Borough population (N=22,010)
Single	12	11	14	13	13	12
Married	35	58	12	22	19	33
Widowed/ divorced	53	31	74	65	68	55
Totals	100	100	100	100	100	100

Source: *Sample Census 1966 County Report for Greater London* (Table 2).

TABLE III. 6

SOCIAL CLASS

Welfare clients compared with borough population
(Percentage distributions)

Social class	Welfare clients (N=296**)	Borough population* (N=119,424)
I and II	5	10
III	45	53
IV and V	50	36
Totals	100	99

*Source: *1951 County Report for Greater London*, Table 27 – General Register Office.

**No evidence available for 4 people.

The social class distribution is also of interest. A comparison of our clients' jobs, or their husbands' jobs, with those of men in their area in 1951 when many were still 'economically active' shows that fewer of the welfare applicants were in professional and managerial jobs and more in semi and unskilled work (Table III. 6).

However, this difference disappears if we compare our sample with the present social class structure of the borough. Selective emigration could be an explanation: a higher proportion of skilled and managerial personnel have left the borough and so by now these old people (most of whom have lived in the area for more than 20 years) resemble those who are left behind.

Housing. A great deal of slum clearance and redevelopment is taking place in the borough; while this may offer hope to some old people in need of rehousing for many it means the loss of the family home they may have occupied most of their lives. Over 50 per cent of the sample (156) had lived at the same address, and an additional 11 per cent (34) in the same district, for more than 20 years. Under-occupation rather than over-crowding was observed: of the 193 clients who lived alone 38 per cent had more than two rooms other than kitchen or bathroom.

Our elderly welfare clients seemed to be somewhat worse off than the other residents in the borough regarding their house tenure.[1] Seven per cent (compared with 14 per cent in the borough) lived in owner occupied houses, and 47 per cent (compared with 38 per cent) in unfurnished privately rented accommodation which in this area is usually older and less well equipped than the local authority dwellings. In other respects too our group of old people appeared to be worse off: proportionately more of them had no hot-water tap, fixed bath or indoor W.C.[1] The latter is particularly hard on old, housebound people. Twenty-seven of the 82 who only had an outdoor lavatory were housebound and very restricted in their mobility. Some of the housing was not adapted to the needs of the elderly; 52 of the welfare clients lived on the second floor or higher without a lift. And although one 79-year-old client living on the fourth floor without a lift remarked that it was 'good exercise', 28 said that they had difficulty with stairs or could only manage them with assistance. Heating facilities were another problem. An open fire was the only means of heating the sitting-room for almost half the old people and over a third had no heating at all in their bedroom. In 44 out of the 118 cases visited in the winter months, the room temperatures were below 60·8°F., the minimum temperature required by the Offices, Shops and Railways Premises Act (1963) for

[1] See Tables 1 and 2 in Appendix 1.

the work places of sedentary workers. Furthermore, only 35 old people lived in a room temperature of 65°F. or above, the minimum temperature to be maintained in cold weather by heating arrangements installed in new local authority houses (H.M.S.O. 1961). It is noteworthy that 23 per cent of the total sample in response to the question; 'Is there any particular expense you find difficult to meet?', mentioned the cost of fuel.

Despite all these shortcomings, when asked whether they were satisfied with their housing 75 per cent answered in the affirmative, though 30 per cent qualified this in some way. Their complaints ranged from inconvenient amenities such as an outdoor W.C., damp, poor state of repair, difficulties with stairs and steps to more personal dislikes such as upsets with the landlord, dislike of the neighbourhood, loneliness and isolation from relatives. A few of the dissatisfied group had recently been rehoused in modern flats, but away from the neighbourhood they knew.

The interviewers made an attempt to assess the housing of each old person in terms of its suitability to their individual needs, using such criteria as the state of repair, whether stairs constituted a problem, and ease of access to the W.C. On this basis 136 of the old people, or nearly half, were assessed as living in unsuitable housing. However, it must be stressed that a considerable proportion of those rated as living in 'unsuitable housing' appeared to be quite satisfied with their environment, living for example in an old terraced house with inconvenient steps and an outside lavatory, in a familiar street, close to relatives and friends. One client probably voiced the feelings of many when she said, 'My memories are here; I don't want to move away.'

Financial Situation. Most of the old people's income came from state sources such as retirement, disability or war pensions and supplementary benefits (Table III. 7). Many had a number of other sources of income, such as sub-letting, work pensions, charity pensions, investments or savings, though most of these sources were small. The table shows that nearly two-thirds of the old people – 197 – were in receipt of supplementary benefits. A few (12) had this as their only income since for various reasons they did not qualify for a retirement pension; but for the large majority it was a supplement to their retirement pension. Twenty-seven or 9 per cent had retirement pensions only. A closer look at their resources showed that 8 might have been eligible for supplementary pensions. For instance, a frail old man of 88 living alone with a dog, paying a rent of £1 7s existed on an income of £4 per week and maintained that this was sufficient for his needs, although he knew that he could apply for supplementary benefits and would be eligible. He lived in a rather dilapidated flat and his neighbours sometimes helped by giving him food. Most of the others whose only source of income was a retirement pension had either some savings or a pension above the minimum, or were living with relatives.

TABLE III. 7

TOTAL SOURCES OF INCOME OF WELFARE CLIENTS

Sources of income	Number of people
Retirement pension only	27
Retirement and supplementary pension only	141
Supplementary pension (without retirement pension)	12
Retirement pension and supplementary pension combined with other sources (e.g. work pension, local charity pension, income from sub-letting, earnings of spouse)	44
Retirement pension (without supplementary pension) combined with one or more other sources (e.g. work pension, disability pension, cash help from family, income from sub-letting)	58
Other sources only (other than retirement and supplementary pension) e.g. war widow's pension, work pension, income from investments or sub-letting	6
No evidence	12
Total	300

It is perhaps noteworthy that among this group of working-class people, many of whom had known real hardship, 82, or 27 per cent had some modest savings – they did not amount to more than £500 in about half the cases. (However, a third did not wish to disclose the actual figure.)

It was difficult to arrive at a reliable estimate of the average income of this group of old welfare clients, since their living arrangements differed and a considerable proportion did not wish to disclose their income. In the circumstances the most meaningful way seemed to be to divide them roughly into four groups: those living in couples, men living alone, women living alone, and those living with relatives or friends. The picture emerging which has to be interpreted with caution is given in Table III. 8.

TABLE III. 8

AVERAGE WEEKLY INCOME OF 238 WELFARE CLIENTS WILLING TO
GIVE THIS INFORMATION*
(1966/67)

Living group	Number questioned	Number responding	Average weekly income of respondents
Living with spouse	36** couples	24 couples	£10 10s 10d (per couple)
Living alone – Men	47	38	£6 11s od
Women	146	121	£6 4s od
Living with relatives/friends – Men	6	5	£6 8s 2d
Women	49	38	£5 7s 4d

*Care is needed in interpreting this table, as people unwilling to reveal their income may be atypical.

**16 couples had both partners in the survey, and 20 had one partner only.

It shows, as other studies have done (Cole and Utting, op. cit., Townsend and Wedderburn, op. cit.), that women living alone are somewhat worse off than men in similar situations.

Asked whether they found it difficult to meet any particular expense, about a third replied 'yes', and special mention was made of fuel (as already noted) and clothing. To the question, 'Do you feel your income is sufficient?', 54 answered 'no', (e.g. 'I could do with a bit more') and the rest were evenly divided between a qualified 'yes' (e.g. 'I manage') and an unqualified 'yes' (e.g. 'I have as much as I want'). Thus on the whole the majority appeared to feel that their income was sufficient. Here one must remember that this is a group of very old people many of whom had given up the struggle for more and were resigned to their fate: 'I know I have not long to live, I make the best of it.' They had experienced much deprivation in their childhood, youth and middle age, which coincided with the appalling poverty around the turn of the century (Booth, 1891) and the period of unemployment during the twenties and thirties. Indeed, a number of them told the investigators that they had never been so well off in their lives. Many of them had brought up large families in poverty and great insecurity; and now at least they were sure of their regular, if limited, incomes.

The Old People's Living Group. We have already mentioned that nearly two-thirds of the old people (193) were living alone. Fifteen per cent lived with their spouse, almost 20 per cent with other members of their family and a few with people who were not related to them (Table III. 9).

TABLE III. 9

LIVING GROUP OF WELFARE CLIENTS

Living group		Number of people
Living alone		193
Living with spouse only		45
Living with other members of family:		55
Spouse and son or daughter	7	
Son or sons	15	
Daughter or daughters	11	
Son and daughter	2	
Son and lodger	1	
Married daughter and family	10	
Other relatives	9	
	55	
Living with non-relatives		7
Total		300

Those who lived alone had significantly more domiciliary services, both meals-on-wheels and home help, than the rest of the group. Not unnaturally they felt more lonely and more depressed than the rest. However, they did not appear to have more unmet social needs, nor did they impress the social work assessors as being more discontented and unhappy than those living with others. Thus, in this small sample of welfare applicants it looks as though living alone did not constitute quite such a hazard or source of unhappiness as is sometimes suggested.

Although old people living with their spouses were on the whole less lonely, they experienced great difficulties when both partners were frail and incapacitated, or even when one of them was very ill or confused and had to be looked after by the other.

The continuing attachment of married daughters to their mothers and their caring attitude towards them, brought out in many recent urban family studies can also be observed in this small welfare sample. While ten of the applicants were living with their married daughters and their families, there was not a single case of an old person living with a son and his family.

Old people who lived with married daughters and their families appeared to experience more stress and interpersonal difficulties than those who lived alone, with their spouses or with single sons and daughters. Friction probably occurred in part because the aged parent was infirm and needed much help and not only because he or she was an interloper, disturbing the customary routine of family life. One of the most extreme examples was a confused and incontinent old man, whose son-in-law and daughter were out at business for long hours and complained that their father soiled chairs and carpets. He was supposed to confine himself to an upstairs bed-sitting-room, but refused to do so, and relationships were at rock bottom when the case was referred. Where an old parent lived with a daughter who was widowed or separated, things worked out more smoothly.

Friction was less evident where an unmarried daughter or son had continued to live in the family home. Eleven old people lived with their single daughter. All these daughters, except two, went out to work while also caring for their mother. Often the working daughter was herself of retirement, or near retirement age: for instance two were in their middle sixties with mothers in their nineties and in both cases the daughters were in poor health. In another two instances daughters had given up work in order to care for the parent at home which meant financial stringency and possibly suppressed resentment. Thus the burden on these daughters was great, though open conflict was less than in those situations where the daughters were married and had families of their own.

In fifteen cases the old people lived with a son. Most sons helped with shopping and household tasks. Some did more, and in one instance a son cared for a chairbound and incontinent mother, dressing her, changing sheets daily, etc., and in another a son gave up full-time for part-time work in order to care for his confused mother. Among these 15 sons we observed a comparatively high proportion of handicapped men. Presumably old people with a handicapped son are more likely to come to the attention of the welfare department and the sons are less likely to marry and leave home. In several cases it was clear that though old and enfeebled, the mother was still a source of support for the handicapped and isolated son.

Social Contacts. Several studies in this country (Townsend, Townsend and Wedderburn, Tunstall, op. cit.) and the international study which extended to Denmark and America (Shanas *et al.*, op. cit.) have shown that on the whole old people in Western industrial society are by no means neglected by their families. Relatives take the lion's share in caring for them when they are ill or incapacitated and keep in close touch with their old folk, despite the ever-increasing social mobility among the younger generation. In the international study 87 per cent of the British sample had been in touch with their children during the 7 days preceding the interview. In our sample, too, children maintained a fairly close contact with their parents. Of the two-thirds who had children alive 77 per cent had seen them at least once, and over half four or more times during the seven days preceding our visit, although a third of the old people did not have a child living within half-an-hour's journey. It is perhaps surprising that this rather incapacitated group should see less of their children than a random sample of ordinary old people in the international study. One of the reasons may be that our group lived in an inner London borough whose population had been steadily decreasing during the last forty years, with the younger families moving out, leaving the older population behind. It may also indicate that those who are referred to welfare departments are somewhat less well supported by their children than those who do not come to the notice of the social services. Most of the children, about 60 per cent, did not merely visit, but also helped their parents with household tasks: many did shopping and other errands for them; in a third of the cases the daughters helped with washing, bringing in or cooking meals for their parents. A considerable number helped with cleaning or in more personal ways – with dressing, bathing or cutting their toenails. A small proportion (14 per cent) were said to help financially or with other extras such as a radio or a TV rental. Neighbours, and to a lesser extent other relatives were also a source of social contact and help. More than two-thirds had held a conversation with a neighbour during the previous week and just over 40 per cent of the old people said that they were receiving help from neighbours which was mainly shopping and to a lesser extent helping with their laundry or cooking meals. Throughout the study the concern and helpfulness of neighbours was very noticeable and it is quite possible that the old people underestimated the help they were receiving from neighbours.

There is some evidence that where an applicant had no children the helping role was to a certain extent filled by a niece or a sister, a neighbour or a friend: of 83 childless old people who lived alone only *one*, an eccentric recluse, had not seen a relative, neighbour or friend during the week preceding the interview.

Asked how many people they had talked to during the previous day, 13 said that they had seen no one. Over two-thirds had seen more than one person and 45 per cent had seen more than two. Thus whilst most of the old people could count on at least one, and some on several interested relatives or neighbours, there was a very small group who could not. Closer scrutiny of the 13 who saw no one did not throw any light on the reasons for this. They were somewhat younger, fewer were housebound or incapacitated than among the sample as a whole. They scored more highly on a composite measure of isolation[1] than the rest of the sample and were somewhat less contented or satisfied, though they did not admit to greater loneliness than the others. Thus they were perhaps not as out-going and lovable as others in the sample. Yet all but one had seen at least one neighbour, friend or relative in the previous week; may be it is not unusual when living alone to see no one on a specific day and it is more meaningful to look at contacts over a week.

Capacity and Attitudes. How did these old people who – as we shall see presently – were afflicted with many major and minor disabilities, manage to look after themselves? In the social interviews we measured the old person's ability to look after himself and his home using Townsend's measures of personal and household capacity.[2] These measures aim at establishing how far the subject can perform the ordinary everyday tasks which enable him to lead a reasonably independent existence. The great majority of the old people were able to dress themselves (Table III. 10) rather fewer could bath without difficulties and practically half the group were unable to cut their toe-nails. Eighty of those who had difficulty or were unable to cut their toe-nails had no one to help them, though 48 would have liked such help. Nearly half could not walk outdoors unaided and over a quarter could not manage stairs at all. Comparing these welfare clients with a national sample in a similar age group (Shanas *et al.*, op. cit.) we find that many more of the welfare clients were moderately or severely incapacitated in terms of

[1] An isolation score was derived from replies to questions about living alone, seeing children, relatives, friends, neighbours and others in the last 7 days.
[2] For a detailed description of these measures see Townsend, P. and Wedderburn, D. op. cit. p. 23.

the functions just discussed: 62 per cent compared with 27 per cent in the national study.

TABLE III. 10

PERSONAL AND HOUSEHOLD CAPACITY OF WELFARE CLIENTS

Welfare client's capacity	Percentage replying (N=300)			
	'Yes'	'With Difficulty'	'No'	No evidence
Walk outdoors	39	19	42	–
Walk indoors	74	25	1	–
Negotiate stairs	28	44	27	–
Wash and bath	76	13	10	1
Dress	82	11	7	–
Cut toe-nails	28	22	49	1
Do light housework	76	13	11	1
Do heavy housework	13	15	72	1
Make a cup of tea	87	4	9	1
Prepare a hot meal	49	24	26	1

As regards household tasks most of the old people were able to make themselves a cup of tea and do some dusting, washing up and a little shopping; but they could not do heavy housework such as cleaning floors and 26 per cent said that they were unable to prepare a hot meal (Table III. 10). Sixty-four per cent of these who had difficulty with heavy housework or could not do it at all had home help or private domestic help, others received help from their families or friends. This still left 28 applicants who said that there was no one to help them, so presumably the basic scrubbing, washing of paint, etc., was never done.

Of the 78 old people who were unable to prepare a hot meal themselves, 29 had meals-on-wheels and the rest were provided for by their own families, friends or neighbours, and only one person said that there was no one to prepare a meal for him.

Since nearly half of our sample were over 80 years old, and over 20 per cent seriously ill, or functionally incapacitated, one would expect them to lead a quiet and restricted life. Like many other old people of their generation they rose rather early, considering that they had little to do during the day. Over half were up by 8.30 a.m. and a quarter before 7.30 a.m. Nearly two-thirds managed to get out at least once a week and over half at least twice a week. Only 52 clients reported that they never went out or were taken out, far fewer than those – 126 – who declared themselves to be housebound. This suggests that they were taken out by relatives or friends or that transport was provided to take them to clubs or day centres.

The main purpose for going out was shopping and collecting the pension. Over a third said they went out for walks. Visits to relatives and friends, hospital and the doctor were also frequently mentioned. Forty-six still went up to the 'pub', 57 of the old people said that they belonged to a club and 53 reported that they had actually attended one the previous week. This is remarkable in view of the sample's age and their disabilities. But there were also those who said that they would 'rather stop by the fire'. At home the most frequently mentioned activities were pottering around, doing some light housework, and preparing food. About half had an afternoon 'nap'. Over half watched TV or listened to the radio and many just sat watching people go by, or thinking about the past. Only a small minority still did sewing, mending or knitting, and about a third did some reading, apart from newspapers which were taken regularly by about two-thirds of the sample. A third enjoyed a 'smoke', but another third had given it up or reduced it, mostly for health or financial reasons. Time passed slowly for quite a number of the old people (31 per cent) most of them living alone; a substantial minority (15 per cent) would have liked a television set, which might have made their lives more interesting. This applies especially to those who live alone, of whom a much smaller proportion had a television set than those who lived with others. Only a few expressed a desire to join a club, but a substantial number (81) would have liked a holiday. (About a third of the old people – 109 – had had a holiday during the last two years.)

Whilst more in our welfare client sample were incapacitated than in a national random sample, one must not ignore the great variability within this group of old people. The sample covered the whole activity range from those who were normally fit and could perform all personal and household tasks without assistance and went out and about, to those who were bedridden and needed help with every aspect of daily living. While the welfare department thus reaches a substantial proportion of very incapacitated people contact is clearly not restricted to the most infirm group of the population.

Physical Health. We have already noted that a considerable proportion of the old people were referred by health agencies and others for domiciliary support in their frailty. It does not come as a surprise, therefore, that nearly a third (29 per cent) of those seen by the physician had been discharged from hospital in the previous year, which is a much higher proportion than had been found in random samples of the population in this age group – 6 per cent to 7 per cent (Townsend and Wedderburn, Parsons 1962, op. cit.). Nearly half said that they had consulted their doctor in the previous month, compared with 37 per cent of a random sample of comparable age.

As has already been said, a detailed diagnostic study was not possible in this inquiry, but enough information was gathered to obtain a fairly accurate picture of the distribution of serious disease and disability among these elderly clients, and of the minor disabilities and discomforts – many of them remediable – which afflicted them.

Surprisingly, anaemia was less common among this group of welfare clients, many of whom were disabled, than among a random sample of old people living in the community in a large county borough in 1962 (Parsons, 1962, op. cit.). Only those aged 75 and over can be compared with this study. Whereas 23 per cent of the women in the elderly population were anaemic, the proportion of anaemic female welfare clients was 10 per cent; and 21 per cent of the elderly men in the county borough study were anaemic, compared with 17 per cent of the male welfare clients.[1] The reason for these differences is not clear. In almost every other respect this group was more incapacitated than random samples of similar age groups in the population.

Only a third (34 per cent) had *no* discernible medical condition or one which, though causing *some* degree of disability, like an arthritic hip-joint, was never likely to be a direct threat to life. Nearly half (42 per cent) were suffering from major conditions which were stable at the time of assessment but which might at some time deteriorate and threaten survival. Old people with cardiac disease in a compensated phase were in this group. And a quarter (24 per cent) were suffering from conditions which were serious and which, without further attention, were thought likely to prove fatal within a year. Among these were people suffering from advanced malignant disease and those

---

[1] Anaemia was diagnosed in men when their haemoglobin was 12·5 grammes or less, in women when their haemoglobin was 12·0 grammes or less (Kilpatrick & Hardisty 1961).

rendered breathless by the slightest exertion on account of cardiac or respiratory disease.[1] The proportion of clients suffering from the severest medical conditions was identical for those under and over 80 years of age. Similar findings emerged in relation to 'functional mobility' (a concept derived from achievement ratings for hand and arm movements and actions involving the trunk and legs): 19 per cent of those aged 70–79 years were rated as poor compared with 20 per cent of those aged 80 and over. These observations suggest that the degree of incapacity is more important than chronological age in determining whether an elderly person is referred to the social welfare services.

Fewer men than women were in poorest health, and in the most restricted category of mobility. This has also been found in earlier studies of random samples in the population (Sheldon, Hobson and Pemberton, op. cit.). Similarly Shanas and her colleagues showed that women aged 70 and over were more severely incapacitated on Townsend's personal incapacity score than men in the same age group. One can speculate that this may be the price women have to pay for their greater ability to survive!

Comparing the medical and social care received by the severely ill and the not severely ill we find that a larger proportion of the severely ill had been discharged from hospital during the previous year (38 per cent compared with 28 per cent), indicating the intractability of some medical conditions at this age. A slightly higher proportion of the severely ill (40 per cent) than of the not severely ill (35 per cent) were attending hospital as out-patients. Information obtained from the general practitioners indicated that roughly equal proportions (40 per cent and 39 per cent) were seen by their doctors monthly or oftener. However, district nurses were attending a significantly greater proportion of the severely ill (20 per cent) than of those not severely ill (8 per cent). We explored whether the district nurses were providing an intelligence service to the doctor on the seriously ill patients with whom he was not in frequent contact. However, this was not so: the district nurse visited less than one-eighth of these cases whilst she attended more than a quarter of the severely ill whom the doctor saw more often.

Apart from the district nurse visits, the severely ill had no more domiciliary services than the relatively fit people in our sample. This

[1] For a detailed diagnostic classification see Table 3 in Appendix 1.

may be because a much higher proportion lived with relatives (52 per cent) than the rest (30 per cent); they also received significantly more visits from their children than the other old people. Consequently the very ill clients were less isolated than the rest of the sample. Twenty-nine per cent were rated as being moderately or severely isolated compared with 40 per cent of the fitter clients. These findings suggest, as other studies have done (Townsend and Wedderburn, Shanas et al., Harris 1968, op. cit.), that families do look after their sick elderly members. Important tasks emerge for the social workers: to ensure that the general practitioner knows about the condition of his patient, and to provide support for these sick clients and their relatives who were caring so devotedly for them.

The social and medical interviews also revealed many minor medical problems, discomforts and disabilities which add a great deal to the burden of old age.

The prevalence of some of these disabilities such as impaired bladder control, and foot conditions requiring chiropody was greater among these South London welfare applicants than in other elderly populations studied.[1] Examination of the feet revealed that 193 of the medical sample (68 per cent) had conditions severe enough to warrant chiropody. Of these 91 were receiving help from a chiropodist or from other sources, but more than half – 102 received no help.

Nearly half of the old people said that they suffered from giddiness. This proportion is similar to that found in other surveys.[1]

Almost a third reported some difficulty in seeing, even when using spectacles. This proportion is again similar to those reporting some difficulty in other surveys.[1] Four old people were registered blind and a further 9 were registered as partially sighted. On testing, visual acuity was found to be adequate for reading lettering of the size of newsprint in all but 21 per cent of the cases and 4 per cent were unable to read print of headline size. A quarter of the old people (whether they had difficulty with eyesight or not) stated they had never had an eye test or had not had one during the previous 5 years, which is a similar state of affairs to that found in other random samples of the elderly.

The prevalence of deafness is known to increase with age amongst the elderly. Nearly one-third of the welfare clients reported that they had difficulty in hearing conversational tones. Similar proportions of the elderly in other areas have reported some degree of deafness.[1]

[1] See Comparative Table 4 in Appendix 1.

When tested, 69 of the welfare clients (24 per cent) were unable to hear two-syllable words spoken in a normal conversational voice. Over a third of these had both ears occluded by wax. Altogether 39 per cent of the medical sample had wax occlusion in their ears (22 per cent in one and 17 per cent in both ears). Thirty-three people had been supplied with an NHS hearing aid but half these had abandoned using them.

Other examples of minor misery were falls, experienced by a quarter of the clients; constipation by a third; and poor or variable quality of sleep by over a third. Fifty-six of the 214 who had dentures were not wearing them. A number of these claimed, nevertheless, to be able to chew their food quite adequately.

These, then, were some of the disabling discomforts and incapacities revealed in the medical investigation. A number of them are undoubtedly irreversable consequences of ageing but many seem remediable to some extent. For instance medical attention of a very simple kind could have relieved some of the deafness and poor sight, and possibly patient explanation and practical advice might have induced more of them to use their hearing aids. In this connection it is worth noting that while nearly half saw their doctor during the preceding month, only 22 per cent claimed to see him regularly and the rest only when specially needed. Thus in the majority of cases such small nuisances as wax in the ear, out-of-date spectacles or foot troubles, may never have been discussed since the consultation was presumably focused on the special complaint for which the old person had gone to the doctor.

Diet. As the diet of the old people is of central importance for their well-being and since it is frequently held that elderly people, particularly those who live alone, neglect their diet, we attempted to estimate the protein intake in our sample. We asked the clients about their dinners during the last week and also their weekly purchases of milk, eggs, cheese and bread. The welfare clients reported buying similar quantities of milk, cheese, bread and eggs as old-age pensioners in the national food survey which was also based on purchases (Table III.11). When comparing welfare clients with the elderly women in the King Edward Hospital Fund's weighed diet study a good agreement was found for milk and eggs (Table III. 11). On the other hand the welfare clients reported more cheese purchases. This was because the sample contained men who ate more cheese than women.

TABLE III. 11

A COMPARISON OF THE AVERAGE WEEKLY CONSUMPTION OR PURCHASE OF
MILK, CHEESE, BREAD AND EGGS AMONG THREE SAMPLES OF OLD PEOPLE

Food	Welfare sample (300 men and women aged 70 and over)	National Food Survey 1966* (1032 households with men aged 65+ and women aged 60+)	King Edward Hospital Fund** (60 women aged 70+, living alone)
Milk (pints)	4·87	5·10	4·5
Cheese (ozs)	3·61	3·33	2·2
Bread (ozs)	34·42	38·86	26·6
Eggs (no.)	4·93	4·56	4·0

Source: * *Household Food Consumption and Expenditure* (1966), Annual Report of the
National Food Survey Committee, H.M.S.O. London (1968).

** *King Edward's Hospital Fund for London* (1965), Report of an Investigation
into the Dietary of Elderly Women Living Alone.

There was a wide range in the amounts purchased by the welfare
clients, those in the top quarter of the distribution buying on average
twice as much as those in the bottom quarter.[1]

Mental Health. Although most of the old people had contacts with
relatives, neighbours or friends and received much help from them,
they still spent many hours alone. We asked them whether they felt
lonely – often, sometimes or never. Probably such a direct question
cannot elicit the complex feelings of loneliness, alienation and disengagement of the very old. Only 39 (13 per cent) of the clients admitted to feeling lonely often; evenings and weekends were mentioned as
bad times for loneliness. More than half maintained that they never felt
lonely.

A rather bigger proportion (155) indicated that they had worries.
Those mentioned most often were illness, housing difficulties, loneliness and family problems. Yet, to the question: 'What do you feel
about your life at the moment?' only 49 (16 per cent) replied that they
were dissatisfied and 165 (55 per cent) felt satisfied.

Since half of those who were severely ill considered their health to be
good or fairly good, we must conclude that these old people are not
given to complaining, at any rate not to strangers in answer to direct
questions and that many were trying to make the best of things. Some
comments point in this direction, for example: 'I struggle on as I am.'

[1] A more detailed account of the results and the methodology of the diet study will be
published separately.

These feelings of resignation were to a certain extent confirmed by a more indirect measure of positive and negative attitudes to the world around them.

On the other hand, feelings of depression and dispiritedness are said to be common among the very old whose life is very circumscribed and who have to face many deaths among their contemporaries and loss of function in themselves. The medical assessor tried to find out the spread of these feelings of depression among this group of old people. He first of all explained carefully what he meant by depression: 'unhappy, down in the dumps, in low spirits, downcast or gloomy'. When he was satisfied after a check that the old person was thinking along similar lines he asked them three questions: 'Do you get depressed nowadays?' 'How often do you feel depressed?', 'How long does the depression last?'

Two hundred and sixty-nine were able to answer these questions and their replies were rated on a graphic scale ranging from 0–5. Since the replies to these three questions turned out to be highly inter-correlated (0·87 to 0·88) an average score was calculated for each person. As Table III. 12 shows, about a third of those who felt able to answer these questions experienced very little depression, and around 20 per cent frequent and prolonged feelings of depression.

We then wondered how these feelings of depression were related to 'depressing' life situations, such as bereavement, living alone, incapacity, isolation and so on. In order to explore this, the depression

TABLE III. 12

DEPRESSION SCORES OF 300 WELFARE CLIENTS
(Based on 3 rating scales)

Depression scores	Number of people
No depression	55
Slight depression	27
Average depression	91
Above average depression	45
Considerable depression	39
Severe depression	12
Interviewed but insufficient evidence	14
Not interviewed	17
Total	300

scores were ranked, with those having the highest scores – the most depressed – at the top and those with the lowest scores – the least depressed – at the bottom. The sample was then equally divided into four, according to this rank order, in such a way that the top quarter had the highest depression scores, the two middle quarters had a central position and the bottom quarter contained the lowest depression scores. These three groups were then compared with other indices (derived from the social questionnaire) which might be associated with depression. The results are set out in Table III. 13.

In relation to most of these indices a clear trend is discernible; the least depressed quarter of the sample appeared to have more favourable experiences, to show more positive attitudes and to need less medical and social work help than those in the top quarter, the most depressed, the rest falling neatly in the middle. The trend only reaches significance level in relation to four variables, which were concerned in some way with what might be termed the 'morale' of the old person: their attitudes to the outside world, their ability to go outside their homes (and presumably meet more people), the social work assessor's rating on their contentment and her judgement on need for casework. This concept of 'morale' emerged as a central one in the experiment, as will be shown in later chapters and (as already indicated) proved to be a sensitive measure of change.

In addition to feelings of loneliness and depression we discovered a fair amount of psychiatric disorder. Thirty applicants were found to suffer from a serious organic brain syndrome and 16 from a functional disorder, as severe as those treated by psychiatric hospitals as inpatients or outpatients.

The prevalence of 10 per cent of serious organic brain syndrome is twice that found in two recent studies among British populations aged 65 and over living in the community (Kay et al., Parsons 1965, op. cit.). These 30 patients were disoriented, showed failure of memory and some wandered away from home, especially at night. Many had difficulties in performing common activities of every day life – 38 per cent were in the most severely incapacitated group in relation to household tasks compared with 12 per cent of the rest of the sample. Their condition was similar to that found in senile dements admitted to psychiatric hospitals.

How did they manage to live in the community? Those who lived with their spouse or with other relatives (18) – a much higher

TABLE III. 13

RELATIONSHIP BETWEEN THE DEPRESSION SCORES AND SOME OTHER
SOCIO-MEDICAL VARIABLES OF 269 WELFARE CLIENTS
(Percentage distributions for each variable)

	Depression scores		
Socio-medical variables	*Least depressed* (N=67)	*Average* (N=135)	*Most depressed* (N=67)
Bereavement less than 3 years ago	22	31	40
No bereavement in the last 3 years	75	67	57
No evidence	3	2	3
Welfare client lives alone	63	64	76
Welfare client not alone	37	36	24
Very socially isolated	10	8	13
Moderately socially isolated	25	34	22
Not socially isolated	64	58	64
Number of people seen 'yesterday' : 0–1	22	25	24
2–3	51	42	42
4 or more	24	31	31
No evidence	3	1	3
Welfare client does not leave the house	9	19	25
Welfare client goes out of doors	91	81	75
Welfare client discontented/unhappy	19	18	55
Welfare client neither content nor discontent	7	18	24
Welfare client contented/fairly content	72	64	21
No evidence	2	1	—
Attitude to outside world: poor	21	32	42
average	37	34	39
good	37	26	15
no evidence	4	8	4
Activity score: low	21	27	24
medium	42	36	33
high	34	36	42
no evidence	3	1	2
Personal incapacity: severe	22	27	34
moderate	19	25	16
fair	33	29	27
none/slight	25	19	21
no evidence	—	—	2

TABLE III. 13 CONTINUED	Depression scores		
Socio-medical variables	Least depressed (N=67)	Average (N=135)	Most depressed (N=67)
'Seriously ill'	13	24	27
'Not seriously ill'	87	77	73
Died during survey	10	12	21
Welfare client and/or relative in need of casework	27	39	49
Welfare client and/or relative not in need of casework	73	59	51
No evidence	—	2	—

proportion than in the rest of the sample – were on the whole lovingly cared for, although their confusion and regressed behaviour – such as soiling and wetting, leaving taps on – proved a great strain to some of the families. Twelve lived alone, which clearly constituted a hazard. Eight of them had either meals-on-wheels, home help, or both and in addition received much attention from their children and neighbours. This left four who appeared to be seriously at risk. They were liable to wander off or did not feed themselves properly, refusing to have meals-on-wheels; they might leave gas taps on or doors wide open in bitter weather.

Specific anxieties such as fear of failing eyesight or decreasing mobility were common and often well founded. In five cases the anxiety was very marked and was accompanied by psychosomatic symptoms which were disrupting the subject's life routine. (One woman aged 77 worried incessantly about her health, despite the fact that she was fully mobile and free from any major medical condition. She was not able to go to sleep for anxiety; she had palpitations, frequent bowel actions, smarting of the eyes and a continual desire to clear her throat.)

Suspiciousness, feelings of hostility or frank paranoid delusions were noted in eight old people. All were living alone and experienced soured relationships with relatives or neighbours, but they were managing to stay in the community when first assessed. Although they harboured some delusions and led very isolated existences these clients were, on the whole, not physically handicapped. They had fewer domiciliary services than the rest of the sample. In spite of this the social work assessors did not consider them to be nearly as much at risk as some of the confused old people with brain syndromes. Their psychosis seemed to have become part of them and their illness did not upset either their way of life or that of others around them.

There were three cases in which depression and other accompanying symptoms amounted to a depressive illness. For example, a widow aged eighty-one was the picture of despair. She complained of feeling depressed, especially in the mornings; she slept fitfully, was constipated and felt that nobody had a kind word for her. She sat looking at the ground shaking her head slowly; her speech was slow and colourless.

Three old people were chronic alcoholics (one of whom had also developed an organic brain syndrome) who presented considerable social problems. Two old people could only be termed 'eccentric'. One, a man of seventy-eight, lived a reclusive life in a tenement flat. He neglected his personal hygiene and lived in great squalor, preferring to sleep on newspapers on the floor, rather than in a bed. He had a certain dignity and independence and did not wish for medical or any other help.

While the prevalence of serious psychiatric disorder (15 per cent) is higher than in random samples of a similar age, we need to remember that most of the old people were in fair mental health and 12 per cent (34 out of the 283 seen by the physician) in very good mental shape. For example: Mr A., an ex-accountant and bachelor, at the age of eighty-seven could hear and see adequately. He was alert and able to answer all the questions related to memory and general knowledge of present events. He showed no signs of depression and to the question 'How do you find the time passes?', replied that he really did not have enough time with two gardens to see to, two lawns to trim and the fires to keep going. This in spite of severely restricted mobility owing to gross osteo-arthritis. He kept up with current affairs and did the *Telegraph* crossword every day. He had applied for meals-on-wheels. His only contact was his neighbour who called in daily; he had outlived all his friends and relatives.

Mrs B. was a childless widow aged eighty-two, an active woman who made a great effort to go out. She attended two clubs regularly and went on many outings. She could hear and see well and was able to answer all the questions testing memory and orientation. She became depressed occasionally, but enjoyed her contacts at the clubs and felt that she always had something to look forward to. She was justifiably worried about her housing conditions, since she had to use an outside lavatory and had no one in the house to turn to in case of illness.

Psychiatric Illness and the General Practitioner. Only about one-third of the psychiatrically ill were said by their doctors to have frequent contact with them. Sufferers from functional conditions were in more regular contact with their general practitioners than those with organic conditions and there was a marked association between frequency of contact and the doctor's awareness of a psychiatric condition. Six of the 8 'functional' cases for whom there was information were said to have seen a psychiatrist, but the general practitioners had not referred *any* of their organic cases for psychiatric advice. Thus only 6 out of the total of 46 patients with well established psychiatric disorders were known to have received specialist psychiatric advice.

Several old people, both among the psychiatrically ill and others, stated that they would not consult their doctors. Thus it must not be deduced that the doctors' unawareness of their patients' problems was due to lack of care or interest. What emerges clearly is that a significant proportion of these applicants for social welfare services required medical attention for psychiatric conditions. Hence an important task for social workers would be to bring these clients' psychiatric conditions to the attention of their medical practitioners and to collaborate with them in any attempts to bring about an improvement in their circumstances.

Services Received and Needed. In addition to the special needs for medical care among the seriously ill (physically as well as mentally) and among those with minor disabilities and discomforts we also examined the needs of the whole group for social support and services of various kinds, as they appeared to the social work assessors. Over two-thirds – 216 (72 per cent) of the old people were already receiving domiciliary services when the assessors saw them (Table III. 14). One hundred and sixty-four had home help for periods ranging from 1 to 9 hours a week with an average of between 4 and 5 hours. About a third – 92 – were receiving meals-on-wheels, most of them five times a week; and 32 were visited by the district nurse whose main help was with bathing and washing.

Allowing for the fact that in 22 per cent of these cases the services had been arranged by the department's welfare officer after the first exploratory visit, it still means that nearly half these old people were already in the 'welfare net' before they became registered clients of the welfare department. This is a very different picture from that presented

TABLE III. 14

WELFARE CLIENTS' REPORTS OF SOCIAL SERVICES THEY WERE RECEIVING AT FIRST ASSESSMENT

Services	N=300	%
Receiving no services	84	28
Receiving at least 1 service*	216	72

Home help	164	(55%)
Meals on wheels	92	(31%)
Chiropody – welfare	69	(23%)
private	13	(4%)
District nurse	32	(11%)
Regular welfare visits (inc. health visitor)	5	(2%)
Voluntary visitors	69	(23%)

*Many clients received more than one service, hence the numbers add up to more than 216 and the percentage to more than 100.

in the international study where even in the highest age group – 85 years and over – only 23 per cent were receiving at least one welfare service.

Most of the old people in our sample expressed satisfaction with the services they were receiving, that is to say they liked their home helps and found them useful and enjoyed the delivered meals. Twenty-six would have liked the home help more often: 'She only has time for the floors. If I ask her to do the windows, she can't do the floors' or 'I suppose she could do the fires if she came every day, but I don't think they can spare her.' Eighteen would have liked the meals-on-wheels service more often.[1] In addition to the statutory domiciliary services over 20 per cent received visits from voluntary workers most of whom were connected with church organizations.

Although 72 per cent of the old people in our sample were already receiving at least one domiciliary service the social assessors uncovered many additional needs – altogether 946 among the 299 interviewed – for services and help of various kinds (Tables III. 15a and III. 15b). Only one person was judged to have no additional needs and the majority had between 2 and 4 additional needs.

[1] At the time of the first assessment the maximum meals-on-wheels distribution was five times a week, but at the end of the experiment this had been extended to a 7-day service.

TABLE III. 15A

NUMBER OF ADDITIONAL NEEDS OF WELFARE CLIENTS

No. of needs for each client	No. of clients	Total needs
0 Needs	1	0
1 Need	39	39
2 Needs	78	156
3 Needs	61	183
4 Needs	59	236
5 Needs or over	57	332
No evidence	5	0
Totals	300	946

Average number of additional needs per person: 3·2.

TABLE III. 15B

ADDITIONAL HELP NEEDED BY WELFARE CLIENTS
AS JUDGED BY SOCIAL WORK ASSESSORS

Type of need		Number of needs
Housing	Rehousing	35
	Sheltered housing	28
	Permanent residential care	14
Domiciliary services	Home help	32
	Meals-on-Wheels	17
	Adaptations	18
	Aids (for handicapped)	16
	'Good Neighbour' service	14
	Library service	12
	Help with garden	3
	House repairs and redecoration	12
Health services	Chiropody	71
	Medical Attention	44
	District Nurse/Bathing Service	16
Community facilities	Club/day centre	75
	Holiday	68
	Outings	12
Material aid	Financial help	22
	Supply of clothes, bed linen, furniture	20
	Loan of T.V.	28
	Loan of wireless	13
Visiting services	Supervisory visits	137
	Casework with welfare client	95
	Casework with relatives	19
	Further casework exploration	41
	Visiting by volunteer	68
	Advice and Information	9
Miscellaneous		7
Total		946

In both the medical and social assessment the need for additional foot care stood out as it does in every recorded survey of an elderly population. A radical expansion of this service would contribute immeasureably towards the comfort and greater mobility of the elderly.

The social work assessors considered that 35 (12 per cent) of the old people needed rehousing, the most common reason being that stairs caused serious difficulty or that the house was in very poor condition. For example, one woman was living in a dilapidated tenement block in which several flats had been closed, there was damp on the wall and ceiling. In a small proportion of cases the old person needed help to move nearer a relative. For instance one old lady on the blind register living alone in a modern local authority flat wished to move to the Midlands nearer to her daughter.

Twenty-eight applicants (9 per cent) were judged to be in need of sheltered housing. They were physically frail, often living alone and apprehensive because they had no one to call on in case of illness. One widow of eighty-two lived alone on the first floor of a terraced house. The outside lavatory was a great inconvenience and since the death of her friend on the ground floor she had no one to call on in case of illness.

Although a quarter of the applicants were attending a club or day centre the social work assessors felt that an additional 75 clients might benefit from the social contact and activities provided in a day centre or club setting. A holiday as a break from the monotony of their lives and as a tonic change was seen as a need for 68 cases. (We noted earlier that many old people expressed a wish for a holiday.)

In most cases it seemed desirable that someone in the department should continue to keep in touch. 'Supervisory' (or review) visits were thought sufficient where a client was managing well with the support of domiciliary services and where the social worker's role would mainly be to ensure that the services still continued to function smoothly and the old person was keeping well. Casework we called a more skilled, though not necessarily long-term form of personal help in which the relationship between client and social worker was of central importance. There were for example some old clients who had lost their spouse and needed help and support through this difficult period of bereavement and readjustment; others who were low and disipirited, it was felt, might respond to a caring relationship. Some in very poor physical health were justifiably anxious and worried about what the future held. There were also a few complex family situations full of conflict in which matters had come to breaking point and in which both the old person and the relatives needed help. In 41 cases (14 per cent) the social work assessors felt that further contact was needed before a full assessment could be made. There was also a small proportion who were refusing to accept any kind of service and who with sensitive understanding might be encouraged to accept domiciliary services and thus to enjoy greater comfort. Some, however, appeared to have deliberately chosen the isolated life of eccentric squalor and were unlikely to respond to a social worker. Voluntary visiting was suggested in 68 cases (23 per cent) where need for more companionship was observed.

Finally it will be seen that only 14 of the applicants were thought to need residential care in a home. Even then 10 of these recommendations were tentative rather than positive and in six cases sheltered housing was suggested as an alternative. All but two of the 14 were over eighty and at least half of them were aware of their need for more permanent and total support, for in answer to the question whether they wanted to go into a home 7 said 'yes', and 2 said they were 'not sure' and only 2 in this group said 'no'. (In the other three cases the question was not asked.) The situations likely to necessitate such a move were as follows: four families who were caring for the old person found the elderly relative too great a burden and were not able to continue; in another case in which the old person lived alone and the son was visiting daily he found the burden too great as well. Another two old persons could not face imminent rehousing and setting up a new flat and felt that it would be more advisable for them to move into an old people's home. Three feared continuing to live alone in case of illness and a few others felt lonely and depressed, in particular two men in their early seventies who wanted to go into a home for reasons of loneliness and depression rather than infirmity.

The 300 old people varied greatly in the number and urgency of their needs. For a minority of the more active clients or those whose families could assume full responsibility for their care, regular contact with the department did not seem necessary, once the required service, say an adaptation, a home help, etc., had been supplied. For most however a social worker seemed to have an important role to play, not least to co-ordinate the bewildering array of services (many administered by different agencies – statutory and voluntary) and to ensure that the many different kinds of help needed, medical as well as social, were obtained and continued to be supplied and used.

Summary. The social and medical conditions and needs of a sample of 79 men and 221 women over the age of seventy, newly referred to a welfare department in south London were assessed by structured interviews.

Most of the applicants, of whom 46 per cent were over eighty, had been resident in the area for more than twenty years; nearly half were living in unsuitable or inconvenient housing in relation to their individual needs. About two-thirds were in receipt of supplementary benefits and though most considered their income sufficient, expenses on fuel and clothing constituted a difficulty for some.

Two-thirds lived alone, 15 per cent with their spouses and 20 per cent with members of their families. Those living alone received significantly more domiciliary services than the rest and did not seem to be more discontented or unhappy than the others in the sample. Much stress and inter-personal difficulties were observed among those living with married daughters and their families; less friction occurred where the old person lived with single, widowed or separated daughters or single sons.

Seventy-seven per cent of the welfare clients who had children alive had seen them during the preceding week and most of the children helped their parents with household tasks and shopping. Neighbours too were a considerable source of contact and very few of the old people seemed to be socially very isolated. They tended to put a good face on things, rarely admitting to great loneliness, dissatisfaction with life or poor health, although a fifth were found to experience frequent and prolonged feelings of depression. These feelings of depression were more marked among those recently bereaved, living alone, housebound or seriously ill.

Considering their incapacity and age many in this sample were still relatively active. Nearly two-thirds got out at least once a week and 25 per cent belonged to clubs. In general there was no evidence that the old people's diet was deficient, and their average consumption of milk, cheese, bread and eggs was similar to that of other samples of elderly people studied.

These old welfare clients were more incapacitated than other random samples in similar age groups studied in the general population of

Great Britain. A quarter suffered from serious disease which constituted a threat to life. Far fewer of these lived alone and they received much care and attention from their families. Many of the old people in the sample suffered from minor disabilities such as difficulties in hearing, seeing, foot trouble, poor sleep, constipation, giddiness, with which they often did not 'trouble' their doctors and which remained unattended.

Ten per cent of the old people were suffering from a serious organic brain syndrome and 5 per cent from functional psychiatric disorders. About a third of these patients were in frequent contact with their general practitioners and the doctors were only aware of about half of these conditions. Only 6 of the 46 patients suffering from serious psychiatric disorders had ever received psychiatric advice.

Half of the sample were already receiving some welfare services before their first contact with the welfare department. The medical and social assessors uncovered many additional unmet needs for social services, medical attention and social casework; most prominent were the usual needs for foot care, housing needs and needs for social recreation, such as clubs and holidays. Most of the welfare applicants were thought to require continuing regular contact with a welfare officer. Only a very few, 14, seemed to be in need of institutional care, half of them because they were becoming too great a burden on their families and half because they could no longer cope with independent life in the community.

References
Abel-Smith, B. and Titmuss, R. M. (1956): *The Cost of the National Health Service in England and Wales*, Cambridge University Press.
Booth, C. (editor, 1891): *Labour and Life of the People*, Vol. 2, Williams and Norgate.
H.M.S.O. (1961): *Homes for Today and Tomorrow*, Report of a Sub-Committee of the Central Housing Advisory Committee (Chairman: Sir Parker Morris, L.L.B.).

PART III

The Social-Work Experiment

4

THE 'SPECIAL' AND THE 'COMPARISON' GROUPS

In the previous chapter we described the social and medical characteristics of the 300 old people who formed the initial sample in the study. As already explained, on referral these 300 clients were randomly but equally allocated to a 'special group' who would receive help from trained social workers and to a 'comparison group' who would be in the care of the department's social welfare officers. In this chapter we shall explore three important questions: first, did the special and comparison groups turn out to be initially similar in essential characteristics? This (as we saw in the introductory discussion) is crucial in order to ensure that any differences in outcome at the end of the experiment were not due to differences at the start. Secondly, what had happened to the initial sample of 300 very old people by the time of the second assessment visit, $10\frac{1}{2}$ months later: how many had remained in the community, or entered an institution or died during the ensuing period? Did those who died or entered an institution differ in any important respects from those who remained in the community? Did these 'losses' affect the two groups equally? And lastly, were the resulting special and comparison groups equivalent at the beginning of the experiment?

Equivalence of Original Special and Comparison Groups
Had the random method of allocation been effective in producing two reasonably matched groups? We compared the two initial groups each containing 150 clients on basic variables, such as age, marital state, sex, social class and living group (See Table IV. 1). On the whole they turned out to be reasonably similar. The table shows that the groups were well matched on age, whether they were living alone and reasonably matched on social class. However, there were 11 per cent more widowed old persons in the comparison group (just below significance

TABLE IV. I

SPECIAL AND COMPARISON GROUPS BY BACKGROUND
VARIABLES AT FIRST ASSESSMENT
(Percentage distributions)

Variables		Special group (N=150)	Comparison group (N=150)
Age:	Under 80 years	56	53
	80 and over	44	47
Marital state:	Single	15	11
	Married	22	15
	Widowed	60	71
	Divorced/separated	3	3
	No evidence	—	1
Sex:	Male	32	21
	Female	68	79
Social class:	I, II, III non manual	11	15
	III manual	37	36
	IV and V	49	43
	No evidence	3	6
Living group:	Lives alone	64	65
	Does not live alone	36	35

level) and 11 per cent more men in the special group (just above the level of significance).

This was unfortunate. If the whole procedure of random allocation had been carried out on a hundred different samples of old people, a result such as this, with more men in the special group, would only have occurred in five samples. The question now arises whether this difference in sex distribution was likely to lead to a distortion in our final results. If the characteristics of men and women proved to be similar then this unequal sex distribution would not matter. A comparison on all the essential measures of the 79 men and 221 women in the initial sample showed that the only important differences between them were that the men as a group were less incapacitated and fewer of them were in the poorest health category, a fact already noted in the previous chapter. However, in spite of this difference in sex ratio, the special and comparison groups did not differ markedly in their physical health. In fact the special group contained a few more seriously ill people. Other detailed analyses failed to show that the difference in the proportion of men and women between the samples was important for the kinds of relationships of interest in the experiment. Nevertheless the difference should be kept in mind.

We then proceeded to test the equivalence of the two groups of 150 old people on all other main variables and criterion measures on which the groups were finally to be compared in relation to outcome.[1] We found that on the whole they were well matched. For example the household amenities of the two groups (fixed bath, indoor w.c., hot-water tap) were similar. The same proportions of each group were living in housing rated suitable or unsuitable by the social work assessors. Just over two-thirds of each group were in receipt of supplementary benefit. Since this relates roughly to a standard level of income, it suggests that on the whole the two groups had a similar financial status. There was little difference in relation to their mental health, though a few more of the special group (4 per cent) had a psychiatric condition.

The two groups were fairly evenly matched on the assessors' judgements of their contentment, on the clients' own expressed attitudes to the world around them and the degree of satisfaction they felt with life at the moment.

As regards social contacts 14 per cent more of those with children in the comparison group had been in touch with their children in the previous week and 15 per cent more had received help from them. This difference (which is statistically significant) it is to be noted, favours the comparison group rather than those for whom the special services were to be provided.

There was hardly any difference between the two groups in the numbers receiving meals-on-wheels and the services of a district nurse at the time of the initial assessment, but somewhat fewer (8 per cent) of the special group had a home help. In the special group also, 4 per cent fewer were attending a club and 5 per cent fewer had had a holiday within the year preceding the initial assessment; so the special group were again, if anything, marginally worse off initially as far as receiving welfare services were concerned.

The groups were also very similar in relation to the number of practical needs each old person was found to have.

Thus, initially the two groups were well matched, with the exception of the greater number of men in the special group.

[1] These detailed tables are available in the Institute's library.

The Situation of the Sample at the Second Assessment
Table IV. 2 shows what had happened to the 300 old people who formed
the initial sample by the time of the second assessment which took place
10½ months later.

TABLE IV. 2

SITUATION OF SAMPLE AT SECOND ASSESSMENT

Situation	Special group		Comparison group		Totals	
	N=150	%	N=150	%	N=300	%
Remained in own homes	111	74	109	73	220	73
Entered residential accommodation	6	4	4	3	10	3
Entered hospital	12	8	10	7	22	7
Died	21	14	27	18	48	16

Of the total, the largest number (220) were still living in the community in their own homes. But around a quarter were not (and this
was to be expected among such an elderly and incapacitated group of
clients); 48 had died, 22 were in hospital and 10 had entered old people's
homes. It will be seen from Table IV. 2 that the numbers dying and
entering hospitals or residential accommodation were similar in both
groups, though four more died in the comparison group. In other
words, 74 per cent allocated to the special group and 73 per cent
assigned to the comparison group of the initial cohort were still in their
own homes when the final assessment took place. Since those who were
in hospitals, in homes or had died do not form a homogeneous group
in relation to their medical and social characteristics, we shall examine
these three groups separately. Broadly speaking, those who were in
hospital more nearly resembled those who died, particularly in their
health characteristics, while those who went into old people's homes
were more like the group who remained in the community.

Those Who Went into Old People's Homes. Not so long ago, for an old
person to ask for help from the local authority welfare department
meant 'the end of the road' and was almost synonymous with applying
'to go into a home'. It is therefore remarkable that only 10 of the
initial 300 applicants had entered an old people's home by the end of
10½ months, and of these two were possibly 'misrouted' and should
have been in hospital; a few others might have been able to manage in

the community if sheltered housing had been available. This comparatively small demand for residential care may be a reflection of the vigorous expansion of domiciliary services for the elderly in this borough. However, it must be noted that we deliberately excluded seven old people who had to be admitted to a home immediately on referral to the department and that at the end of the experiment ten clients (5 in the special and 5 in the comparison group) were on a waiting list for residential accommodation.

Since the number entering an old people's home were so small we cannot draw any general conclusions about their characteristics, but a few observations may be of interest.

Those who went into permanent residential care were older as a group than those who remained in the community (7 out of 10 were over 80 years compared with 43 per cent). Four out of 10 were men (compared with 2·6 among the community group). Seven were widowed and 3 single. Five of the 10 were living alone. In the case of at least 3 of the 5 living with relatives or friends, difficulties in their relationships appear to have been a precipitating factor. Seven out of 10 were living in housing rated unsuitable by the assessor (compared with 43 per cent of those who remained in the community) and in each case stairs were a problem for the old person. Four of these 10 people also expressed dissatisfaction with their housing, although the houses of the 10 were not worse in general amenities than that of the clients remaining in the community.

Five of the 10 said, at the first assessment interview, that they had considered the possibility of going into an old people's home, compared with only 1 in 5 of those who stayed in their own homes.

The initial assessments indicated little difference in degree of infirmity between the 10 who went into old people's homes and those who stayed in their own homes. For instance, the two groups did not differ in their ability to get about or their capacity to perform everyday tasks or in the severity of their medical condition as rated by the medical assessor. This is in contrast to the Government Social Survey's findings (Harris 1968, op. cit.) that, in nearly all the local authority areas studied, more of the residents of old people's homes had difficulty in performing various everyday activities than a general sample of retirement age. However, our numbers are very small and ours was a special sample of welfare clients who were already more incapacitated than is usually found in random samples of similar age. This presumably explains why the 10 going into old people's homes were no more infirm than those staying at home and suggests that additional social problems tipped the balance. In other respects too the 10 as a group did not differ from those at home except that they tended to be somewhat less contented. For instance, 6 of the 10 said they were often or sometimes lonely, and four were rated as discontented or openly unhappy by the assessor; in both cases this proportion is more than among those remaining at home and was related to their unhappy personal relationships.

Thus in this tiny group it looks as though social reasons, both situational (housing) and personal, rather than incapacity in itself, are associated with entering a home.

Those Who Went into Hospital. Twenty-two old people had to be excluded from the 'before' and 'after' comparison on the social measurements because they were in hospital at the time of the second assessment. However, all of them were seen by the social work and medical assessors. The reasons for their exclusion were not only that many of the questions about their present social condition and needs did not apply while they were in hospital, but practically all these clients were so ill and confused that they could not respond to a detailed interview. Whenever a client was known to be in hospital on the date of the second assessment, we waited a month in case he was able to return home, before conducting an interview in the ward and excluding him, or her, from the experimental sample. In the physician's opinion fourteen of those in hospital at the time of the second assessment were unlikely ever to return to the community.[1] The rest he considered would only be able to leave hospital if special domestic arrangements could be made to cope with their serious illness. Since equal proportions of the old people in the special and comparison groups (8 per cent and 7 per cent, see Table IV. 2) entered hospital it is unlikely that their exclusion introduced a bias into the findings.

We now want to examine whether these 22 clients in hospital differed in any important respects, when first seen, from those who remained at home. They were slightly younger and fewer lived alone, which may

[1] It should be noted that these 22 were not the only clients in the sample who *ever* went into hospital during the course of the experiment. Thirty-three went into hospital and returned home; only one-third of these were found to be seriously ill on second assessment.

suggest that old people who are ill are more likely to go and live with someone else who can care for them. (This corresponds with the findings in the last chapter that proportionately more seriously ill and incapacitated clients were living with others.) Unlike those who went into homes – many of whom lived in unsuitable housing – welfare clients going into hospital were if anything slightly better off in this respect than those remaining in the community. This may be related to the fact that they lived more frequently with their children in more modern housing. A fairly high proportion, 7 of the 22, had considered the possibility of going into a home. They were on average more sick, less mobile and less active when first seen than those who remained in the community. Nearly half had been assessed as severely ill (compared with 14 per cent of those who remained at home); 13 were housebound and 9 could not manage stairs at all or only with assistance. 'Activity scores' based on their activities during the previous week were lower. It is of interest that although many were sick and incapacitated they did not seem to be in frequent touch with their doctor: just over half of them – the same proportion as among those who remained at home – had seen their doctor within the past month, and a third had not seen their doctor in the previous three months. Five suffered from a severe psychiatric condition, which is a higher proportion than in the group who remained in the community.

Considerably more of those entering hospital had domiciliary services when first visited: 17 of the 22 had home help, 10 had meals-on-wheels and 4 had district nurse visiting. This is the more noteworthy when one bears in mind that fewer of those who went into hospital lived alone. Another favourable feature noted was that they saw their children more frequently than did those who remained in the community. Possibly for all these reasons the social work assessors did not find any more unmet needs among the hospital group than among those remaining at home.

One might expect this group of sick old people to be more depressed, unhappy and lonely than a more active group but in fact the differences were small in these respects.

Taking all these observations together it appears that the very sick and infirm went into hospital mainly for medical rather than for social reasons, as they had more contact with their children and more services than the other clients in the sample. One could also speculate that their hospitalization may in part have resulted from the favourable conditions in which they lived: their families and the social services saw to it that they had hospital care when they needed it.

Those Who Died. The largest group of old people who did not remain in the community until the time of the second assessment were the 48 who died, comprising 16 per cent of the original sample of 300. Table IV. 3 shows some of the more important ways in which those who died differed from those who did not when first seen.

TABLE IV. 3

DIFFERENTIATING SOCIAL AND MEDICAL CHARACTERISTICS AT
1ST ASSESSMENT OF WELFARE CLIENTS WHO DIED COMPARED WITH
THOSE WHO SURVIVED TO 2ND ASSESSMENT
(Percentage distributions)

Characteristics	Dead ($N=48$)	Living ($N=252$)
Marital state		
Single	4	15
Married	10	20
Widowed	81	62
Divorced/separated	4	2
Suitability of housing		
Very suitable/suitable	35	58
Unsuitable/detrimental	63	42
No evidence	2	—
Mobility		
(1) Able to move outside building	31	62
Confined to building	67	37
No evidence	2	—
(2) Able to climb stairs:		
Freely unaided	8	31
With difficulty	42	43
Only with assistance	15	4
Not at all	33	21
No evidence	2	—
Activity score		
Low	35	23
Medium	33	38
High	19	27
Very high	2	9
No evidence	10	3

TABLE IV. 3 CONTINUED

Characteristics	Dead (N-41*)	Living (N-242*)
Severity of medical condition		
No or very little illness	7	38
Stabilized medical condition	34	44
Serious illness threatening life	59	18
Haemoglobin level		
Norman haemoglobin	78	91
Low haemoglobin	17	7
No evidence	5	2
Breathlessness		
Not breathless on exertion	41	69
Breathless on exertion	56	31
No evidence	2	1
Depression		
Very little depression	17	25
Some depression	39	49
Serious depression	34	22
No evidence	10	4

*Only 283 of the sample of 300 were seen by the physician.

Significantly more of them were widowed (81 per cent compared with 62 per cent) and fewer single (4 per cent compared with 15 per cent). Very many more were living in housing considered unsuitable. This is probably connected with the fact that they were somewhat older, had lived longer at their present address than the survivors (26 per cent compared with 12 per cent of survivors had lived 40 years or more at the same address), and occupied older-type accommodation. On the initial assessment the group who died were on average less mobile than those who survived. Sixty-seven per cent of them were housebound and 48 per cent could not manage stairs at all or only with assistance (these percentages for the survivors were 37 per cent and 25 per cent respectively). Another indication that those who died were less active was their much lower ratings on the activity scores (Table IV. 3).

Only 41 of the 48 who subsequently died were originally assessed by the physician. Fifty-nine per cent – 24 people – were judged to be suffering from conditions which threatened survival, compared with only 18 per cent of the survivors, a highly significant difference. Significantly more of them had a low haemoglobin level and suffered from breathlessness on exertion. More of those who died suffered from feelings of depression, but this difference was not significant.

Few differences emerged in the social characteristics between those who subsequently died and the rest of the sample. The proportions of those who lived alone were similar. They did not receive more visits or help from their children, but they did have more home helps and district nurses visiting than those who survived. There was no difference in the number of unmet needs seen by the assessor and there was little difference in their attitudes to life.

Equivalence on First Assessment of Final Special and Comparison Groups
Two hundred and twenty of the initial sample of 300 old people were still living in the community in their own homes at the time of the second assessment. Very little information was obtained at first assessments about six of these, because of illness or confusion, and they were excluded from the final analysis. Thus there were finally 214 old people – 110 in the special group and 104 in the comparison group, which was comfortably within our target of 100 people in each group. These 214 people were the subject of the main field experiment and it is therefore important to examine these two groups of 110 and 104 people who remained in the community, to see if they were as well matched at the beginning of the experiment as the initial sample.

In the main they were well matched, as can be seen from Tables IV. 4 and IV. 5 giving the basic background features and many measurements, which will be used to compare the two groups with respect to the outcome of social work. At this point it is only relevant to mention those aspects in which the groups differed.

The differences found in the initial comparisons regarding sex and widowhood became slightly more marked (37 men and 63 widowed people in the special group compared with 18 men and 72 widowed people in the comparison group). The other significant differences between the two groups were that the comparison group had had more visits and more help from children when first assessed and that this group saw their general practitioner more often at home than at the surgery. Since the comparison group did not contain any more severely ill people this difference is surprising, unless it ties up with the fact that 12 per cent more old people in the comparison group were restricted to their homes. It is unlikely that this difference between the two groups would have any effect on the outcome of the experiment.

TABLE IV. 4

SPECIAL AND COMPARISON GROUPS OF FINAL SAMPLE BY BACK-
GROUND VARIABLES AT FIRST ASSESSMENT
(Percentage distributions)

Variables	Special group (N=110)	Comparison group (N=104)
Age		
Under 80 years	60	55
80 years and over	40	45
Marital state		
Single	14	13
Married	25	15
Widowed	57	69
Divorced/separated	4	2
Sex		
Male	34	17
Female	66	83
Social class		
I, II, III non manual	11	17
III manual	36	34
IV and V	51	45
Unclassifiable, no evidence	2	4
Living group		
Lives alone	67	66
Does not live alone	33	34

TABLE IV. 5

SPECIAL AND COMPARISON GROUPS OF FINAL SAMPLE BY IMPORTANT
SOCIAL AND MEDICAL VARIABLES AT 1ST ASSESSMENT
(Percentage distributions)

Medical variables		Special group (N=101*)	Comparison group (N=96*)
PHYSICAL HEALTH	No or very slight illness	41	35
	Stabilized Medical Condition	43	51
	Serious illness threatening life	17	14
MENTAL HEALTH	Evidence of severe psychiatric condition	13	11
	No apparent evidence	87	89
	Very little depression	24	28
	Some depression	50	52
	Serious depression	24	20
	No evidence	3	0

Social variables		Special group (N=110)	Comparison group (N=104)
HOUSING	Very suitable/suitable	57	58
	Unsuitable/detrimental	43	42
FINANCIAL SITUATION	Receiving Supplementary Pension	69	70
	Not receiving Supplementary Pension	31	30
	No evidence	0	1
	No difficulty in meeting expenses	51	63
	Difficulty with 1 expense	40	33
	Difficulty with more than 1 expense	5	1
	No evidence	4	3
	Income sufficient	33	41
	Income barely sufficient	42	40
	Income not sufficient	25	17
	No evidence	1	1
SERVICES RECEIVED	Has home help	48	55
	Does not have home help	52	45
	Has meals on wheels	27	31
	Does not have meals on wheels	73	69
	Visits doctor	65	45
	Doctor calls	34	55
	No evidence	1	0

*Only 283 of the sample were seen by the physician.

(TABLE IV. 5 CONTD.)

Social variables		Special group (N=110)	Comparison group (N=104)
DIET	Low score	21	23
	Medium score	46	39
	High score	29	36
	No evidence	4	2
NEEDS	0–1 Need	32	35
	2 Needs	23	27
	3 Needs	23	23
	4 Needs	14	10
	5 Needs	9	5
	Average	2·4	2·1
SOCIAL CONTACTS AND HELP	No one seen yesterday	5	5
	1 person seen yesterday	20	19
	2 persons seen yesterday	25	31
	3 persons seen yesterday	25	18
	4 or more persons seen yesterday	24	26
	No evidence	0	1
	Average	2·7	2·7
	No contacts with children in past seven days	32**	15**
	1–3 contacts	24**	22**
	4–9 contacts	18**	32**
	10 or more contacts	26**	31**
	Help given by children	43**	76**
	Occasional or restricted help given	19**	5**
	No help given by children	38**	19**
ATTITUDES	Attitude to outside world good	25	26
	Attitude to outside world fair	34	37
	Attitude to outside world poor	34	32
	No evidence	6	6
	Satisfied with life at the moment	58	63
	Mixed feelings	21	19
	Dissatisfied with life at the moment	19	15
	No evidence	2	2

**Only applies to those with children, e.g. 74 and 61.

95

Mention should be made at this point of three items, quite highly inter-correlated, which will be shown later to emerge as a 'factor' in the component analysis (see Appendix 2). These three items concerned sufficiency of income, difficulty in meeting expenses and the social class of the old person. Although the two groups did not differ significantly on the items taken individually, the special group was significantly 'worse off' on the combined 'factor', in having more difficulty in managing on their income and containing more old people of lower social class.

Two of these three significant differences between the groups – the contact with and help from children and the financial factor – clearly favour the comparison group.

A comparison of the two groups on the assessors' global and more 'clinical' judgements regarding the client's general contentment the prevalence of personal problems and the degree of their need for social work shows them to be fairly well matched in these respects (see Table IV.6). This is of interest as it indicates that the social workers' tasks in each group would be of comparable proportions. The clients in the special group were judged to have a few more difficulties than those in

TABLE IV. 6

SOCIAL WORK ASSESSORS' GLOBAL ASSESSMENT OF WELFARE CLIENTS
(Percentage distributions)

Assessments		Special group (N=110)	Comparison group (N=104)
CONTENT-MENT	Contented/fairly contented	57	52
	Neither contented nor discontented	17	20
	Discontented/openly unhappy	25	26
	No evidence	1	1
PERSONAL PROBLEMS	Pronounced	17	12
	Moderate	41	44
	Slight	28	32
	None	14	12
INDICA-TIONS FOR SOCIAL WORK	Considerable	19	13
	Moderate	41	46
	Slight	35	38
	None	4	4
	No evidence	1	0

the comparison group: 5 per cent more of the special group had pronounced personal problems and 6 per cent more were assessed as having 'considerable' need for social work.

Thus despite the 25 per cent loss in both groups (which we expected in this age group and allowed for in the design of the study) the final special and comparison groups were still reasonably similar. Where they differed significantly in important respects, the differences on the whole worked to the disadvantage of the special group, thus increasing the challenge to the professionally trained social workers.

5

THE SOCIAL WORK

We have shown that the clients in the special and comparison groups who were the subjects of the experiment were on the whole similar in their physical and social characteristics except that there were more men in the special group. If anything, random allocation seems to have worked slightly to the advantage of the comparison group (Table IV. 5).

Before we can go on to consider the outcome of the social work in the two groups we need to determine whether there were any real differences between the social work 'input' in the special and comparison groups.

Organization of Social Work
As soon as the social work and medical assessors had seen a client, the senior social worker in whose area the client resided was informed whether the case had been assigned to the special group or should be retained on their district caseload. If the case was to be passed on to the project workers, this did not as a rule present any difficulties, as the local authority social worker had paid only one preliminary visit.

Neither the project social workers nor the department's social workers knew what questions the assessors were asking in their interviews, nor did they ever learn what the assessors' opinions were about particular cases. The assessors worked from a separate office at the headquarters of the welfare department. They never discussed any cases directly with the local authority social workers or the project social workers. Any message that had to be conveyed – because the assessors, for example, had come across an urgent need or request – was passed on to the appropriate social worker through the administrative secretary of the project.

The borough was divided into four sub-districts headed by a senior social worker for purposes of the welfare service. Each of the project social workers was responsible for special group cases in two of these districts. They, like the local authority social workers, worked under the general direction of the senior social workers in their areas, consulting them mainly on administrative and policy matters, whenever the need arose. The distribution of the study cases within the four districts and their allocation to the special and comparison groups are shown in Table V. 1. It will be seen that the distribution was fairly

TABLE V. I

CASLOADS OF SOCIAL WORKERS IN SPECIAL AND COMPARISON
GROUPS IN THE FOUR AREAS OF THE BOROUGH

District	1st Assessment				2nd Assessment			
	Special group		Comparison group		Special group		Comparison group	
	No.	%	No.	%	No.	%	No.	%
Area 1	51	34	50	33	41	37	33	32
	78				61			
2	27	18	24	16	20	18	18	17
3	29	19	25	17	18	16	17	16
	72				49			
4	43	29	51	34	31	28	36	35
TOTALS	150	100	150	100	110	99	104	100

balanced between special and comparison groups and also that the project social workers each had a comparable caseload, one of them working in areas 1 and 2 and the other in areas 3 and 4. Area 1 was the poorest and most densely populated part of the borough with the highest referral rate (see Table V. 1), which explains the slightly higher caseload of the project worker in areas 1 and 2. Area 4 was a much larger, widely spread district.

The project social workers had their own separate office on the top floor of one of the area welfare departments, since the experimental design required as little contact as possible between them and the social workers in the comparison group. The experimental conditions also imposed certain other restrictions: for example, they were not able to participate in the area case conferences as inevitably there would have been a good deal of interchange on casework methods, use of resources, etc., and, since the project workers were more highly trained, the local authority social workers might have been tempted to use them in a consultative capacity. In short, there would have been a good deal of 'contamination': the project social workers would have learnt about the social work methods of the local authority workers and vice versa. The project social workers had their own regular weekly case discussions with the director of the study who is herself a trained caseworker.[1]

The project social workers did take part in administrative staff meetings in their respective areas, for although they were on the payroll of the National Institute they worked under the general direction and jurisdiction of the authority's chief welfare officer; for the duration of the experiment they constituted additional staff in the welfare department. Throughout, they had an easy and friendly relationship with their colleagues. To begin with both project workers spent one month in an area office working alongside the local authority workers to familiarize themselves with the area, its resources and with the rules and procedures of the welfare department. Neither of them had ever worked in a welfare department before. Considering this, and the very short period of acclimatization, it is remarkable that no important administrative mishaps occurred throughout the two-year period of the experiment. The only very minor slip happened when on one or two occasions the local authority workers mistakenly visited old people who had been assigned to the special group. The remarkably smooth working of this complex experiment, which required the active collaboration of many different people, is an impressive testimony to both the personnel of the welfare department and the project social workers. The implications will be discussed in the concluding chapter.

Some Characteristics of the Social Workers
Forty-one local authority social workers dealt with the 104 cases in the comparison group over the period of twenty-one months' field work. Their age and sex distribution is shown in Table V. 2. It will be seen that their age range was very wide and that the large majority were women. Table V. 3 relates their age to the qualifications they held. Although a number of the local authority social workers were professionally qualified as home teachers for the blind, or as health

---

[1] This meant that the director kept herself as separately as possible from the assessment side of the study. She never saw any of the assessment questionnaires until after the completion of the fieldwork. Any 'supervision' required by the assessors was carried out by the statistician. The director was only consulted in emergencies or when policy decisions had to be made, which were very rare occasions.

TABLE V. 2

AGE-SEX DISTRIBUTION OF 41 LOCAL AUTHORITY SOCIAL WORKERS
CARRYING 104 CASES IN COMPARISON GROUP

Age group in years	Women	Men
20 —24	9	–
25 —34	8	6
35 —44	3	–
45 —54	12	–
55 and over	3	–
Totals	35	6

TABLE V. 3

QUALIFICATIONS OF 41 LOCAL AUTHORITY SOCIAL WORKERS BY AGE

Type of qualification	Age groups					Totals
	20–24	25–34	35–44	45–54	55+	
Basic university Social Science qualification	4	2	1	1	–	8
Basic university qualification & Home Teacher for the Blind Cert.	–	–	–	1	–	1
Degree/diploma (unrelated)	1	2	–	1	–	4
Other professional training	–	2	2	4	2	10*
Home Teacher for the Blind Cert.	–	1	–	1	1	3
Diploma in Sociology	1	1	–	1	–	3
Overseas social-work qualification	–	1	–	–	–	1
None of the above	3	5	–	3	–	11
Totals	9	14	3	12	3	41

* 5 were S.R.Ns. followed by health visitor training,
  1 was a registered mental nurse,
  1 was an occupational therapist,
  1 was a teacher,
  1 was a housing manager,
  1 had taken a Salvation Army training course.

visitors, and many of them had long experience of welfare work (often supplemented by short courses), only one worker, who took a diploma course in a European country held professional social work qualifications.

It is noteworthy that 6 of the 8 who had taken a basic social science course were under thirty-five and that most of the 23 local authority social workers under thirty-five were hoping to take a professional social work training.

The two workers appointed by the National Institute for Social

Work Training were both psychiatric social workers. One was a married man in his late twenties and the other a single woman in her late forties. The former had had two years' experience in community care of the psychiatrically ill and in child guidance and the latter had long years of experience in all branches of mental health work and also in family casework. Thus the two workers were of very different age and experience and their approaches to the work were also different in some respects: for instance, the young male worker was particularly interested in behaviour therapy and social action, whilst the other worker was more committed to the psycho-dynamic approach in casework.

The male worker was inclined to see more problems per case than his colleague. Being a warm-hearted young man holding radical views who had to deal with many elderly women some of whom were very spinsterish and timid, he not unnaturally found 52 per cent of his clients 'difficult' to help. His colleague, on the other hand, an outstandingly tolerant and patient woman, only thought 12 per cent of her clients were 'difficult' to help. And while he thought that 20 per cent of his clients were 'very responsive' in their attitudes to him, his colleague thought that 39 per cent were 'very responsive'. At the other end of the scale, the young male worker felt that 10 per cent of his clients were hostile, whilst his female colleague did not acknowledge any active hostility from any of her clients. It is of course quite possible that these very elderly women when faced with a modern young man were more difficult and hostile in their attitudes and generally less responsive than to a maternal-looking, middle-aged woman social worker who could enter more naturally into their feminine preoccupations.

It is of great interest that, in spite of the very evident differences in breadth of experience, approach and in the theoretical framework these two social workers were using, the outcome of their cases was strikingly similar whenever we compared them. This could be due to a variety of reasons: to common principles in their training, to their close contact during the experiment in which they influenced each other's work greatly, and to their regular joint case discussions with the director.

These discussions ranged very widely, beyond the specifics of individual cases to a consideration of methods in relation to different types of cases, the actual and potential role of a wide variety of community resources and the ideology and content of social work with the elderly in the context of a welfare department.

Considerable differences were also noted in the approaches and activities of the various social workers in the comparison group. Some workers were quite young and inexperienced, though they may have had a university education, others had long years of experience and training in related professions, supplemented by extramural studies. At the one extreme were social workers who only recognized the most obvious problems and did mainly routine or emergency work; at the other extreme were social workers with mature judgements, acute perception of clients' attitudes and needs and subtly differentiated ways of helping people. Visiting patterns also varied and were not necessarily related to the size of their caseloads. Some workers with very heavy caseloads were able to see their clients fairly frequently; others did not manage more than 3 or 4 visits in a year.

Whatever the differences *within* the two groups of social workers – and they were clearly considerable – there was one clear cut difference *between* the social workers in the special and comparison groups. The former both had a basic social science qualification followed by a professional training in social work, while in the comparison group only 22 per cent had completed a basic social science course and none had a professional social work qualification (except possibly the one worker with the Continental diploma).

The second fairly important difference was that in the comparison group 63 per cent of the clients had more than one worker during the $10\frac{1}{2}$ months of fieldwork; in the special group every client had the same social worker throughout.

Thirdly, the social workers in the special group had more time than the social workers in the comparison group. They certainly had far fewer cases than their local authority colleagues at the beginning and towards the end of the fieldwork period. During the middle phase of the experiment they each had about 75 cases which is still considerably less than the caseload of around 120 carried by their colleagues in the welfare department. However, three other factors have to be considered: the workers in the special group had to cover a much larger area. They each ranged over two whole districts while their colleagues often had only a number of adjacent streets to look after, which enabled them to visit many clients during one day. Secondly, the social workers in the special group were new to work with old people; they were both strangers in the area and comparatively unfamiliar with the administrative machinery and usages of a welfare department. In consequence, they did not know the area nearly as well as most of their colleagues in the welfare department and inevitably took longer in finding the right resources and arranging practical details. By definition all the cases of the project social workers were of recent origin, while the caseloads of the local authority workers also contained long-standing routine cases. Although the time factor is important it looks, as we shall show later, as though the amount of time spent does not by itself account for success or failure in particular cases.

Difficulties of Measuring 'Input'

In clinical trials in medicine one is reasonably sure of the different kinds 'of treatment given to the experimental and control groups. Usually the patients in the experimental group receive a drug whose pharmacological components are known and the other patients receive either a different drug or a pseudo-drug, a 'placebo'. As a rule the therapists are not aware which patients receive which drug and thus even their psychological set towards the patients cannot be influenced by the knowledge of the medicine they are administering and their belief or disbelief in it. In a field experiment in social work we cannot ever adopt this 'double blind' method of the clinical trial, i.e. the therapists themselves not knowing whether the patients they are treating are in the experimental or control group.

Indeed we have to accept the fact that the project workers knew that by definition their cases were the 'special' ones and that their work would be scrutinized. This probably enhanced their motivation which was all to the good, since the workers themselves, their skills and their relationships with the clients were the 'medicine' we set out to test. The local authority workers on the other hand did not know which of the new cases had been assigned to the comparison group, since many referrals were excluded because they did not meet the criteria laid down for inclusion in the study, and several times intake was stopped altogether because of pressure in numbers. The local authority workers were only able to identify clearly the cases assigned to the special group as they had to hand them over to the project social workers. Furthermore, the study cases formed a very small part of the local authority workers' big caseload; there was ample evidence in the final interviews with them, and in their extraordinary uniform visiting patterns over the two-year experimental period, that they had not been aware of any impending examination of their work with particular clients.

Most social work experiments carried out so far have experienced formidable difficulties in describing concretely, let alone in measurable terms, the nature of the social work treatment given to both the experimental and the control groups (Meyer et al., Brown, op. cit.). The investigators usually use such terms as 'casework' or 'group work', or they give impressionistic accounts of the work done, or describe the work carried out in the experimental group in considerable detail, giving practically no information about the work in the comparison group (Blenkner et al., 1967 op. cit.). The outstanding exception is the experimental study of different forms of casework treatment of family problems by the Institute of Welfare Research of the New York Community Service Society. Here careful measurements were applied to the casework in all the treatment groups (Reid 1968, Reid and Shyne, op. cit.).

In our study an attempt was made to categorize and to a certain extent measure, the social workers' assessments of their cases, their prescriptions and their social work 'treatment' by asking the workers in both groups a series of simple questions about each case immediately after the independent social and medical reassessment had taken place at the end of the experimental period.

These interviews, in addition to factual information, gave us some insight into the local authority workers' ways of handling cases and into their attitudes, which could then be compared with those of the project social workers. The first set of questions was aimed at discovering the social workers' assessment of the case in terms of the problems observed, the degree of need for social work and the kind of help indicated at the beginning of the case. Questions followed about the extent and nature of the social work done, the number of visits and interviews that had taken place, what other agencies had been contacted, what practical services had been rendered and what kind of psychological help had been attempted. We then tried to explore the relationship between the client and the worker in very simple terms and to obtain the workers' own assessment of the degree of success they thought had been achieved in each case, asking also for supporting evidence for these judgements. Finally, we inquired what problems their clients still presented. The measuring devices used were simple and crude and probably only gave a very rough idea of the workers' perception of their clients and the actual helping process, but they have the advantage of being reasonably objective and it was possible to carry out independent checks on some of the statements made about the social work done. These crude measurements brought out striking and highly significant differences between the two sets of workers.

Perceptions of Problems and the Need for Social Work

Tables V. 4a and b show interesting contrasts and similarities in the social workers' perceptions of their clients' problems. The distribution of the problems (Table V. 4a) was on the whole similar, that is to say both sets of workers thought that the majority of their clients suffered

TABLE V. 4A

INITIAL PROBLEMS SEEN BY SOCIAL WORKERS
(Percentages)

Problems*	Special group (N=110)	Comparison group (N=104)
Physical disability	92	86
Housing	29	33
Financial difficulties	11	3
Poor home conditions/inability to cope	5	6
Burden on family	10	5
Social isolation/loneliness	45	47
Difficult interpersonal relationships	20	9
Mental and emotional disorders ⎱ Worries and anxiety ⎰	40	24
Miscellaneous	6	4

*Most clients had more than one problem.

from physical disabilities, that almost half were seriously isolated or lonely and that about a third experienced housing problems.

There was one striking difference between the two groups. The project social workers saw mental and emotional disturbances in 40 per cent of their clients whilst the social workers in the comparison group assessed these difficulties among 24 per cent of their clients. It is likely that training and experience in the mental health field had sensitized the psychiatric social workers to emotional difficulties; but we also recall that the medical assessor had discovered a few more cases of psychiatric disorder among the special group, although the difference was not of the same order (14 per cent in the special and 11 per cent in the comparison group).

The social workers in the special group identified significantly more problems per case than their colleagues in the welfare department, the average being 2·6 compared with 2·1 in the comparison group (Table V. 4b). Again the distributions are not markedly dissimilar, for instance over a third of the clients had two problems in both groups and about

TABLE V. 4B

NUMBER OF PROBLEMS SEEN PER CLIENT

Number of problems	Special group (N=110)	Comparison group (N=104)
1	17	27
2	40	41
3	31	30
4	17	6
5	4	0
6	1	0
7	0	0
Average no. of problems	2·6	2·1

28 per cent had three problems in both groups. But it is at the extreme ends of the distribution that the two sets of workers diverge. The project social workers diagnosed four or more problems in 22 cases whilst their colleagues only diagnosed 6 such cases. These differences may in part be independent of the social workers' perceptions, since it will be remembered that the clients in the special group were somewhat worse off in several respects (more psychiatric disorder, more serious illness, less visiting and help from children). However, the social work assessors did not see any substantial differences in the number of problems experienced by clients in the special and comparison groups, the average being two for both groups.

The fact that the special group social workers recognized more problems than the social workers in the comparison group tends to confirm one of our hypotheses, namely that the professionally trained workers would recognize more problems than experienced, but partially trained social workers. Similar pointers emerged from Jefferys' survey of social work in Buckinghamshire (Jefferys 1965).

From an intensive study of a 10 per cent sample of case records in both groups it appeared that the project workers recognized depression hidden under a brave face more readily. They were able to spot subtle but disturbing family situations which may not have been clearly visible: for example, in families where members were either over-protective, not allowing the old person any independent activity of their own, or where relatives were denying any strain and refusing domiciliary services, or when relatives felt guilty about letting their spouse or parent go into hospital.

Differences also became apparent in the social workers' estimate about the degree of need for social work (Table V. 5). The social

TABLE V. 5

'NEED FOR SOCIAL WORK' SEEN BY SOCIAL WORKERS IN SPECIAL AND COMPARISON GROUPS AND 'INDICATIONS FOR SOCIAL WORK' SEEN BY SOCIAL WORK ASSESSORS*
(Percentage distributions)

Social workers' judgements			Assessors' judgements		
Need for social work	Special group (N=110)	Comparison group (N=104)	Indications for social work	Special group (N=110)	Comparison group (N=104)
Very great	33	16	Considerable	19	13
Moderate	45	60	Moderate	41	46
Minimal	22	24	Slight/none	39	41
			No evidence	1	—

* Unfortunately a somewhat different terminology was used by the assessors and the social workers; thus the observations are probably only roughly comparable. It will also be noted that the assessors used a 4-point scale and the social workers a 3-point scale.

workers in the special group thought that twice as many of their clients (33 per cent) were in very great need of social work. The social workers in the comparison group on the other hand more often judged the need for social work to be moderate (60 per cent) than the project social workers (45 per cent). The assessors also judged that more people in the special group had considerable need of social work than in the comparison group. But the difference is much smaller than the difference between the two sets of social workers. In general, the social workers in both groups saw more need for social work than the assessors (Table V. 5). This is probably due to the fact that the assessors had to base their evaluation on one visit while the caseworkers were judging the initial situation with hindsight at the end of 10½ months of social work when problems had had a greater chance of becoming visible.[1]

Although the objective indications are that the special group had marginally more problems and were possibly in greater need of social work than the clients in the comparison group, we feel justified in concluding that the project workers' perceptions of their clients' problems and of their need for social work were different from those of their colleagues. This difference may be associated with their training, much of which is directed towards discovering problems and towards more differentiated diagnostic thinking.

Does this mean that the social workers in the special group recognized more problems which really did exist or that they 'found' more problems, whether they existed or not? This is a very difficult question which cannot be answered definitively. As already indicated many of these judgements or 'insights' refer to the level at which problems are perceived, taking one's evidence both from cues which may not always be obvious and from the here and now of the interaction between clients and social workers.

As will be seen later, the social workers in the special group did by no means ignore practical problems; indeed they gave significantly more practical help to their clients than their colleagues in the comparison group.

The Social Workers' Prescriptions
The social workers' prescriptions for their clients also varied in expected directions (see Table V. 6). While the department's social workers most commonly felt that their clients needed social services and supervisory visits, the project social workers more often saw a need for social services and casework with the old person or their relatives, or with both. This difference was very great and highly significant statistically – 58 per cent in the special group against 23 per cent in the comparison group.

The intensive study of a 10 per cent random sample of cases suggests that these prescriptions were in fact followed. Whilst in the comparison group services were sensitively offered and administered and the clients' right to choice respected and no effort spared to make life more

---

[1]Another explanation may be the different scales used. One was a 4-point scale with the extreme rating as 'considerable', the other a 3-point scale with the extreme rating as 'very great'.

TABLE V. 6

TYPE OF SOCIAL WORK NEEDED AT REFERRAL AS SEEN BY SOCIAL
WORKERS IN SPECIAL AND COMPARISON GROUPS
(Percentage distributions)

Type of social work	Special group (N=110)	Comparison group (N=104)
Supervisory visits only	12	16
Services only	5	4
Services and supervisory visits	22	45
Services and casework with old people	33	15
Services and casework with relatives	3	1
Services and casework with old people and relatives	22	7
Casework with old people only	4	6
Casework with relatives only	o	o
Casework with old people and relatives	1	6

tolerable and comfortable, more subtle resistances or perplexing family situations often remained unrecognized and unexplored. The workers in the special group laid equal emphasis on practical help and the provision of services, but at the same time they paid much attention to their clients' subjective experiences and feelings. For example, in one of the sample cases the local authority social worker in her initial visit was quite satisfied that an elderly wife, because she declared herself ready to do so, was able to look after her bedridden husband unaided; the social worker in the special group to whom the case was allocated recognized – on his first visit – the importance of this burden on the wife, her divided feeling about this and planned his work with this in mind. As already mentioned, the social workers in the special group were more likely to spot covert depression, and in these cases they provided opportunities for talking about the loss and feelings of despair before helping the old person to pick up the threads again and to venture into new social contacts, say in a club or on holiday.

Another interesting difference was in the varying ways in which the social workers in the special group combined practical and psychological help, 'advocacy' and casework.

For example, recognizing that an old lady was totally discouraged, feeling useless with no contribution to make, the social worker would find small ways of helping her to regain some sense of worth and use, if only by learning again how to do some simple knitting. Relatives would be drawn into the helping process, by example or by imaginative suggestions and encouragement. In one case the social worker, having obtained a wheelchair and meeting much reluctance on the part of the relatives to take their mother out in it, wheeled the client out herself for a while. At the same time she gave the embittered daughter opportunities for ventilating her feelings; eventually, without being asked, this daughter took over from the social worker. On other occasions relatives or others in the clients' social network were helped towards a more responsive attitude to the client, leading to practical action – fitting grab rails or decorating his house. Such helpfulness had previously been blocked by a mutually uncomprehending and almost hostile attitude between the client and others. Another situation the social workers were able to recognize was that of over-protection and the smothering of the old person's active self, not only by relatives but by over-eager, kindly intentioned neighbours, who in this way were contributing to the old person's inactivity and regression. Here the social worker's job was to reinforce what capacities and independence still remained without antagonizing the 'protectors' or depriving them of their caring functions. The psychiatric social workers also engaged in active advocacy, speaking on behalf of the incapacitated old person, upholding their rights and legitimate wishes when occasion demanded. For example, one old lady, having been turned down for an almshouse on account of a potentially disrupting psychopathic son, had her case reconsidered and obtained the almshouse as a result of such active advocacy. Concurrently the social worker engaged in casework with both son and mother in order to minimize any disturbance the son's behaviour might cause and to strengthen the mother's resolve to maintain her independence.

Frequency of Visits
It is extremely difficult to summarize adequately the complex activities which we call social work. No claim is made that the quantitive comparisons which follow do justice, especially to the casework relationship and the more intangible aspects of this highly personalized form of social service. Yet unless we break down the social work activities into their component parts and attempt to quantify them, we shall not be able to compare the 'input' in the two groups. We will then have to resign ourselves to talking in the vaguest terms about

'casework' or 'social work' and will be unable to put our finger on what it is that distinguishes more effective from less effective social work.

The first quantifiable aspect of social work is the frequency of contact with the old people and their relatives. As Table V. 7 shows the project social workers paid on average twice as many visits to their clients as the workers in the comparison group. Fifty-eight per cent of

TABLE V. 7

NUMBER OF VISITS MADE BY SOCIAL WORKERS IN THE SPECIAL AND COMPARISON GROUPS
(Percentage distributions)

Number of visits	Special group (N=110)	Comparison group (N=104)
0 − 1	0	6
2 − 3	4	13
4 − 5	7	25
6 − 7	12	22
8 − 9	20	16
10 − 11	11	3
12 − 13	8	5
14 − 15	13	3
16 & over	26	8
Average no. of visits per client	14·1	7·1

the clients in the special group were visited once a month or more, whereas this only applied to 19 per cent of the comparison group. The reasons are manifold and probably related to the size of the caseload. As mentioned before, the project social workers never carried more than 76 cases each, while the caseload of the local authority social workers was around 120, and in times of staff shortages more than that.

If we plot the social workers' visits in relation to the growth and decline of their caseloads over the 21 months of field work a suggestion arises that other factors, principally motivation, enter into the picture. The project social workers paid many more visits to their first 20 cases (average 23·2) than to the clients referred during the middle period of the experiment when they were carrying their maximum load (average

9·7 – less than half). Although the frequency of their visiting picks up again as their caseload decreases towards the end of the experiment (for cases were handed back to the welfare department after reassessment at 10½ months), it never reaches the initial average number of 23 visits for a similarly small caseload, but stays around 14. Many influences may be at work, but motivation is certainly one of them. Clearly the keenness, the excitement, the desire to prove one's worth will not be as strong at the end as at the beginning of such a novel experience. The caseworkers' thoughts were turning towards the new jobs they were entering after leaving the project, they were spending more time writing up their notes and reading the literature. They were also more experienced and possibly did not expend effort any more where it clearly would not bear fruit.

In contrast, in the comparison group where the social workers were not aware of the part they were playing in the experiment and where the project cases only formed a minute part of their caseload (most workers had no more than 3 to 4 project cases), the frequency of visiting hardly fluctuated at all over time. The average number of visits paid to the first 20 project cases was 5·75, in the middle period it was 5·95, and at the end 6·25.

Another interesting phenomenon is the very different distribution of the number of visits paid in the special and comparison groups (Table V. 7). In the special group, with the exception of four cases who received 3 visits or less, we find an almost equal proportion of clients being visited between 4 and 7 times and between 12 and 15 times, with a higher peak between 8 and 11 visits. In the comparison group there is a great concentration of clients – about half – who were visited between 4 and 7 times. These different distributions and the intensive study of the random sample of cases, suggest that in the comparison group pressure of time and possibly also lack of recognition of more subtle casework problems cause this kind of division between 'ordinary' cases and 'demanding' cases.

A visit once in two months could be managed in the majority of 'ordinary' cases which required a certain amount of supervision and support, while an intensive effort could only be expanded on those few clients who made a lot of demands either because of the severity of their problems, or because emergencies arose. It looks as though the workers in the special group were able to exercise more choice over how they were going to distribute their efforts. Thus they paid comparatively few visits to those old people who were managing fairly well without them, well supported by their family or neighbours, or to those who laid great store by their independence and who did not really feel the need for support by a social worker. They paid a fair number of visits to old people who required some supervision because of their infirmity or in other precarious circumstances. They concentrated their efforts not only on those who made constant demands or faced emergencies but also on those with more hidden needs, who could make use of patient and intensive casework, or where they could see possibilities of enriching lives by extending social activities and role functions. For instance they did intensive visiting in an effort to help people over their bereavement; ('after my husband died she kept coming', p. 176). In another case the social worker offered an uncritical and truly supportive relationship to a lonely and alienated alcoholic who would be considered 'unhelpable' by many a social worker. The social work included personal introduction to a club and mediation when the client got into difficulties there; encouragement of neighbourly contacts was another facet of the social-work effort which entailed many ups and downs and disappointments. In yet another case the project social worker embarked on a regular contact with an old man shut up in his room with his fantasies, gradually enriching his life, first by visiting him, then by providing visits from an occupational therapist and lastly by introducing him to a club and arranging a holiday. This old man was by no means openly unhappy or neglected by his relatives to begin with and could easily have been written off as 'managing adequately' in his room, and as not requiring any additional services.

Practical Help and Contacts with Other Agencies
In general the aim of social work with these old people was, wherever possible, to ensure their well-being and physical comfort, to reinforce, and to add to the roles which, however small, they could still perform, in an attempt to enhance their feelings of worth and identity. The skill in social work with the elderly may well consist in being sensitive to the possibilities and to the limits of the client. This means that the social worker has to find the right balance between accepting the legitimate 'closing of accounts' (a process that has been called 'disengagement') on the one hand and encouraging social contacts and other enriching influences that are still possible, on the other (Cumming and Henry 1961, Cavan 1962).

TABLE V. 8

PRACTICAL HELP RECEIVED AND ATTEMPTED
(Percentages)

Type of help	Received		Attempted but not received	
	Special group (N=110)	Comparison group (N=104)	Special group (N=110)	Comparison group (N=104)
Housing:				
Rehousing	6	5	14	6
Admission to residential home	1*	1*	7	12
Domiciliary services:				
Home help	22	6	8	7
Meals on Wheels	15	2	5	5
Adaptations	14	2	6	2
Aids	30	23	3	2
Voluntary visiting/ Voluntary help	32	8	25	6
Personal assistance	14	10	2	0
Decoration of home	8	2	7	2
Occupational therapy	5	4	6	1
Health services:				
Chiropody	16	13	3	2
District Nurse/bath attendant	6	6	2	2
Medical attention/ Hospital admission	31	10	5	3
Community facilities:				
Club/day centre	35	13	35	27
Holiday	23	14	31	13
Outings	21	10	8	4
Transport/escort (e.g. to club)	25	7	3	2
Material aid:				
Christmas parcel	34	21	3	0
Financial help	17	9	5	1
Provision of material goods	5	7	0	0
Extra nourishment	16	2	4	2
Other	4	1	0	1
Average No. of items of help received	3·9	1·8		

* One client in each group was temporarily admitted to a private home.

The first aim, of ensuring physical comfort and well-being, entails a great deal of practical help and liaison with all kinds of social and medical services. As can be seen from Table V. 8, the social workers in both groups arranged for much practical help which these elderly clients needed as shown by the initial assessments. This is not all: on the right-hand side of the table we see a fairly formidable list of practical services which the social workers attempted to provide for their clients but which did not come to fruition for various reasons. The clients themselves may not really have wanted or needed them, a typical example being a carefully arranged holiday from which the elderly person withdrew suddenly revealing that after all alternative arrangements had been made to spend the holiday with relatives. Or after visiting a big and somewhat noisy club, the client would decide that he preferred to stay quietly in his own home. In some instances the services after much searching and negotiating were not available: rehousing adapted to the old person's individual needs was a conspicuous example, inability to find a really suitable voluntary visitor was another. (This happened in 25 per cent of the cases in the special group.) Lack of transport at convenient times was yet another frustrating influence.

In some cases lack of opportunities for more specialized and intellectually stimulating activities in clubs and day centres contributed to the failure to draw the old client into a socially satisfying group, especially among men and middle-class clients. There also seemed to be room for smaller and more individualized activities for old people who, though wanting to get out, were not 'clubbable' in the conventional sense. Finally the services required could be so much delayed – adaptations were a regrettable example – that the time of greatest need had passed when the alterations could be carried out; the relatives might have rigged up a device, or the client was by now chairbound.

These many attempts which did not come to fruition indicate that the provision of practical services for the elderly is not always a simple act of arranging for meals-on-wheels or for organizing transport to a club, or providing a wheelchair. It can involve a great deal of preparatory work and of reaching out to the old people. This applies particularly to this generation of old people who, having experienced great deprivation, tend to be resigned to their decreasing mobility, growing isolation and restriction of their life space and may prefer to leave things as they are. However, there were also very demanding old people, never satisfied by whatever services were provided. Such attitudes may also have sprung from personal and general deprivation.

The low expectations of many of these old clients formed a barrier which most social workers found difficult to overcome. The social workers in both groups showed a deep respect for the human dignity and right of choice of their clients, never trying to over-persuade them, if all they wanted was to be left alone. In the special group the case-workers and the director had many searching discussions on these themes, particularly in relation to very disturbed or eccentric clients who involved the social workers in certain dilemmas of conscience. For example, the eccentric old gentleman who lived the life of a recluse in great squalor and discomfort, insisting on sleeping on a pile of newspapers and refusing all offers of bedding or any other help. He cooked on an open fire and would not see a doctor about his septic foot. He only consented to see a social worker at very infrequent intervals when he would engage in general conversation, never allowing the social worker to get anywhere near his personal problems.

The questions we asked ourselves were: were we endangering the life and safety of this client and others because of the obvious hazards of the pile of newspapers catching fire; were there any ways in which we could induce him to accept medical attention and a more comfortable and less isolated existence? However, the more eager the social worker was to help him and to enter his world the more the old man kept him at bay. Having made sure that the authorities did not consider compulsory action necessary in view of the potential fire and health risks, the social worker continued his occasional visits on the client's terms which did not lead to any change in his circumstances. It was difficult to resign ourselves to our inability to bring about any change and to accept as valid this man's choice as to how he was going to live.

There were other potentially dangerous situations which could threaten the survival of clients. For instance when clients did not feed themselves sufficiently to maintain life, were lying seriously ill in bed refusing to call a doctor, or if they were cooking on an open fire with arthritic or trembling hands. In these situations the social worker may have to make decisions which go against the expressed wishes of the client, practically ignoring the much-discussed 'principle of self-determination' in the interest of the old person. This is particularly true in cases of severe mental confusion.

Despite all these difficulties of making resources available and acceptable to their clients, one glance at Table V. 8 shows that the workers in the special group rendered substantially more help to the old people in almost every respect, than did their colleagues in the comparison group. On average they provided twice as much practical help per person (3·9 items compared with 1·8); and while they arranged for four or more items of practical help in over half the cases, this only applied to a quarter of the cases in the comparison group. One of the most striking differences relates to attendance at clubs and day centres which was achieved in 22 per cent more of the special cases. The provision of transport and escorts to clubs also differed markedly between the groups. This not only involved official transport; the workers themselves would often, in order to ease their clients into a club and give them confidence, accompany them for a few weeks before letting them make their own way either on foot or by local authority transport. (It should be noted that both the project social workers had cars in contrast to most of the local authority social workers; this was essential because they covered a much bigger territory.)

We note a substantial difference in the amount of voluntary visiting and other voluntary help used in the special group in contrast to the comparison group. If the cases in which the project social workers tried but did not succeed are added to those in which they were successful in introducing a volunteer, we see (Table V. 8) that they considered voluntary help appropriate in over half of their cases. Both the social workers themselves and the director of the study were particularly interested in enlisting volunteers to enrich the lives of their old clients. The welfare department, in addition to collaborating with existing voluntary associations, had a special scheme for organizing voluntary help, which at that time drew mainly on schoolchildren for its source of supply. This worked out quite happily in some cases, but in others the visits of schoolgirls, for example, rather late in the day when the old people felt tired, were not always convenient. Nor did the children always see the point of 'just visiting' when there were no chores to be done. Consequently the two social workers, looking after the special group, turned to other possible sources of help. This partly explains the project workers' very much greater contact with voluntary agencies (Table V. 9), 43 per cent compared with 12 per cent in the comparison group. The Red Cross, Salvation Army, Rotary Club and many other possibilities were explored in order to find more mature volunteers for the old person. Some suitable people were found, though this achieve-

TABLE V. 9

CONTACT WITH OTHER AGENCIES
(Percentages)

Type of agency	Special group (N=110)	Comparison group (N=104)
Organizer of volunteers	51	12
Club organizer	47	17
Home Help Service	34	33
Meals-on-Wheels organizer	24	27
Local authority Housing Department	30	23
Miscellaneous local authority departments	9	3
Ministry of Social Security	32	13
Old People's Welfare	21	7
Voluntary agencies (Red Cross, Salvation Army, W.R.V.S., etc.)	43	12
General practitioner	50	31
Local authority Health Department (Other than Home Help)	32	19
Hospital social worker	22	8
Other hospital services	14	3
Geriatric/psychiatric consultants	9	0
Dentist	5	1
Optician	8	2
None	1	12
Miscellaneous	22	8
Average no. of contacts per client	4·5	2·2

ment was by no means proportionate to the effort expended. On the whole, the great trouble taken to involve volunteers did not bear the fruit we had hoped and some of the reasons for this and suggestions for the future are discussed in the last chapter.

The other marked difference revealed both in Tables V. 8 and V. 9, is the greater concentration of the project social workers on medical attention, on liaison with general practitioners, consultants and other health authorities. Medical attention or hospital admission was facilitated in 31 per cent of the cases in the special group and in only 10 per cent of those in the comparison group. Contact with general practitioners was established in exactly half of the cases in the special group compared with a little less than a third in the comparison group. One of the reasons for the much closer collaboration with medical agencies on the part of the project social workers may have been that they were both psychiatric social workers, used to team work and consultation with medical colleagues. Several doctors in the area expressed surprise at the way in which the project social workers discussed problems and at their intensive casework activities. They intimated that they had been used to look to the welfare department for the provision of services rather than casework. This contact with general practitioners and hospital specialists led to fruitful combined efforts in several cases, for instance collaboration to provide specialist treatment or social support on discharge from hospital. The workers also experienced a certain amount of resistance and apathy towards active therapeutic intervention with the very old. Some general practitioners felt that in view of the patient's age and infirmity it was hardly worth while to try a hearing aid, or arrange for a functional assessment, or to refer a depressed old person to a psychiatrist for therapy. The social workers were not very successful in overcoming this type of resistance and often felt the need for a geriatric consultant to be available to the welfare department's social work staff, as is visualized in the recommendations of the Seebohm Report.

Another sphere in which the social workers in the special group were particularly active was finance, checking wherever necessary whether their clients were receiving their correct supplementary allowances or benefits to which they were entitled, for instance rate relief. They would obtain discretionary grants from the local office of the Department of Health and Social Security in suitable circumstances – for special needs such as clothing, bedding, removal expenses and for special equipment such as safety stoves. Occasionally they would raise financial grants from voluntary sources. Collaboration with the Department's local officers was on the whole good, and if approached with a well-reasoned case they were prepared to use their discretionary powers. Occasionally the social workers in both groups encountered the problem of the old person's own depressed standards and their obstinate refusal to apply for supplementary allowances to which they were entitled. One such case is described in Chapter III, p. 55.

It is also worth noting that the workers in the special group took up the housing problems of a fifth of their cases, but achieved little within the ten months at their disposal. Extremely inconvenient accommodation which lacked adequate facilities for even an able old person was not improved in a number of cases despite the hardship it caused to the old people concerned. Some clients were offered rehousing in another part of the borough, but the housing authority's failure to plan on a neighbourhood basis meant that locally rooted old people did not feel able to accept these offers and were not accommodated. However, the social workers succeeded in forging good links with the housing authorities. They discussed the particular personal needs of their clients who, within the very extensive redevelopment plans of this borough, would have to move soon. For instance they would stress the life-line to a neighbour who might call daily and do their shopping, and the desirability of moving them together; or the importance of ground floor accommodation with a small patch of garden for an old widower whose life centred on his garden. The housing authorities were interested and open to suggestions of this kind. Occasionally one of their officers would follow up these discussions with a personal visit to the client with resulting reassurance.

Another contrast between the two groups was the extent to which extra nourishment was provided. (Table V. 8). It will be remembered that old people whose protein intake seemed to be below a certain level were notified to both sets of workers in order to see whether they were able to exert any influence on their diet. The project social workers took a special interest in this aspect of the experiment. They discussed diet and meal patterns, occasionally providing Complan[1] themselves to begin with. They also tried to interest relatives in the dietary aspects and suggested ideas for improving the diet of their elderly parents or spouses. The social workers in the comparison group (who were also notified of the poorly nourished clients in their caseloads), seemed to have done little about it, apart from routine inquiries and ensuring, in suitable cases, that meals-on-wheels were regularly supplied.

The greater provision of home helps and meals-on-wheels for clients in the special group (Table V. 8) may be related to their having less contact with, and help from, their children than the clients in the comparison group (see Table IV. 5, p. 95).

Provision of residential accommodation constituted only a small part of the social workers' activities in both groups, since only 10 clients of the original sample went into an old people's home. This kind of help is not referred to in Table V. 8, as those who went permanently into a home automatically dropped out of the final sample.

[1] Complan, made by Glaxo, is a protein, mineral and vitamin supplement in powder form.

Psychological Help

Looking at the old people and their social situation along three dimensions: firstly their age and degree of infirmity, secondly their capacity to cope with their handicaps and thirdly the environmental support available – we could discern roughly three groups with differing needs and demands for social work.

1. The ordinary ageing person who may or may not be incapacitated to some extent whose *handicap is made tolerable* by either a constructive, optimistic attitude on the part of the old person or by a good supporting network of family and friends, and/or social services.

2. The severely physically handicapped old person whose *infirmities and dependency create problems for him and his environment*, however good the old person's morale may be and however adequate the social support.

3. The old person with a marked emotional or mental disturbance or a long-standing *personality disorder who creates considerable problems* for the people who look after him, even with social work support.

Among the first group of the ordinary ageing person, who were minimally handicapped, of good morale, and well supported by family, friends or social services, the amount of casework or psychological support required was minimal. In these situations, once contact had been made and any necessary services provided, the social worker acted as a supervisory link, or co-ordinator of services, ensuring from time to time that the services were still functioning adequately. The social worker was always prepared to intervene as soon as an acute illness or an accident, the loss of a relative or a friend caused a crisis. These kinds of cases – in the estimate of the project social workers – constituted about a third of their caseload. In their opinion these clients did as a rule not require the services of a fully trained caseworker.

Among the second group of clients, amounting to nearly half, the aim of social work was to provide physical and psychological comfort, often in the shape of aids and adaptations which contributed to easier mobility and safety. Occasionally the social workers encountered reluctance among these old people to accept appropriate help or to admit that they needed any assistance at all, that for instance they could not manage an open fire any longer, should have a bath rail to avoid accidents, and so on. In these circumstances, the social worker's first job was to help the clients to accept that their growing infirmity necessitated help from others. Detailed and definitive advice often followed. It will be seen from Table V. 10 (p. 125) that the project social workers thought that they had given advice in almost two-thirds of their cases. Complex activities then had to be set in train in collaboration with many other agencies, with doctors, hospital personnel, with those who provide domiciliary services which often had to be adapted to the special needs of a very enfeebled or disabled old person. In these cases the social worker's co-ordinating role became crucial and required much skill and patience. Last, not least, the social worker was often involved with the patient's family or with the supporting neighbours or friends, who were shouldering much of the day-to-day care, strain and responsibility. One thinks here particularly of elderly spouses who wear themselves out lifting their aged companion, trying to cope with incontinence, and attending to their many small needs, refusing to admit defeat. The social worker had to use much tact and sensitivity in tackling such situations. Having clarified needs and convinced the relative that help was needed, this help had to be offered in such a way as not to deprive the spouse of his supporting role, avoiding at all cost making him feel useless or superfluous or even neglectful. Such a situation became even more precarious when the aged relative had to be admitted to hospital, since there was always the dread that this may be his last journey. Relatives often reproach themselves for depriving their spouse or parent of the comfort of dying in their own home. There were also the reverse situations in which relatives were eager to push the ailing old person into hospital. Those left behind could then find many convincing reasons for their action in an attempt to cover their feelings of guilt.

Sensitive support and acceptance of the differing ways in which people cope or fail to cope with strain was part of the casework with such families.

Among this group of very disabled and sometimes depressed and dispirited old people were some whose situation could not be changed, whatever efforts were made and where the social workers were limited to holding a watching brief. Even this could sometimes provide a source of psychological support. There were also those who by very patient effort could gradually be stimulated to venture out again into the outside world by means of a holiday or attendance at a club or just by visiting a neighbour instead of the neighbour always coming to

them. At first the social worker often had to listen to many reminiscences and much inward-looking fantasy. When the social worker
was sufficiently in touch with the old person's inner world he sometimes was able to discover where the present outside world could still
impinge and become a pleasurable experience. We have already quoted
two such examples in the special group (p. 114) of patient exploration
and building up of a relationship preparatory to other enriching
experiences.

Very difficult casework problems were encountered in dealing with
seriously confused old people and among clients with other mental and
emotional disorders, some of them lifelong, and certainly not remediable in advanced old age. This group constituted about a fifth of the
caseload. To help the seriously confused client close collaboration with
other social and medical services was needed, but often rendered very
difficult by the clients' inability to co-operate and by his irrationality.
Intensive, regular follow-up, deliberate reaching out, sometimes in an
almost authoritarian manner, toleration of aggression and 'ingratitude'
and preparedness for any kind of emergency were some of the ingredients of casework among such deeply disturbed clients. Examples of
this demanding kind of social work were found in both groups.

Clients with long-standing personality disorders, hardly distinguish-
able from ingrained neurotic disturbances posed quite different
problems. The first need was to recognize these disorders and to set
realistic limits on the help that was possible. For even in old age such
people can be aggressive, subtly manipulating, sabotaging services; or
they can be passive and dependent, surrounded by a great deal of help
which can be almost deliberately concealed from the social worker
who may expend much energy in befriending such people, trying to
introduce them to volunteers and clubs, only to find that they are
already getting a full share of support. Help was also rendered difficult
because sometimes these disturbed old people lived in disturbed
families, or long years of personal and material deprivation had
engendered negative or unreasonably demanding attitudes.

Straddling all these groups were the problems of depression and loss
which afflict so many old people who come to the attention of the
welfare services. We saw in Chapter IV, Table 4, that over 20 per cent
of the clients were found to be severely depressed and about 50 per cent
moderately so. Depression in the elderly may appear as disorientation,
accompanied by neglect of home and self. It was as a rule very difficult

to get these depressed old people to consult their general practitioner, for they did not recognize their state as a remediable medical problem; they accepted their misery with resignation as something which was inevitable in old age.

The social workers in the special group tried to help these people by listening, letting them talk about their past and present relationships if they wanted to. This kind of ventilation was intended to ease their feelings of despair and isolation before any attempt was made to help them to reintegrate themselves into any still existing social network of relatives and friends or to find new opportunities for them. In several cases help towards reintegration into a more active life was not necessary at all once the bereaved person had emerged from his period of mourning and depression; he then appeared to be perfectly capable of finding his own way. Hardly any examples of this kind of work were found in the comparison group.

In this connection it is worth noting that the project social workers said that they had encouraged ventilation of feelings in nearly three-quarters of their cases, whereas the social workers in the comparison group only acknowledged this kind of casework activity in less than half their cases (Table V. 10).

TABLE V. 10

PSYCHOLOGICAL HELP GIVEN
(Percentages)

Type of help	Special group (N=110)	Comparison group (N=104)
General support	88	73
Ventilation of feelings	74	41
Advice	63	33
Clarification of real situation	52	18
Discussion of problems in present relationships	34	9
Discussion of problems in past relationships	23	1
None of these	4	4
No evidence	0	2

Similarly the social workers in the special group thought that they had discussed problems in past and present relationships with over a third of their clients, while this only applied to 10 per cent of the cases in the comparison group (Table V. 10). The project social workers also reported a much greater use of their clarifying role, sorting out problems and situations with clients' relatives and as mediators between clients and other agencies.

Differential Social Work
It is clear that these different types of clients required very different kinds of casework and we have tried to give a descriptive account of social work in varying situations in which quantitative measures played a minor part. We also attempted to look at clients' problems and the amount of help provided in a more quantitative way: Did those who were considered to be greatly in need of social work receive more help than those whose needs were thought to be more moderate or minimal? In order to answer this question we took as our baseline the assessors' initial judgements, whether the clients' needs for social work were 'considerable', 'moderate' or 'slight'. We see from Table V. 11 that in both groups, but markedly so in the special group, most effort in terms of average number of visits, contacts with other agencies and items of practical help, was expended among those with 'considerable' need for social work, less on those who had 'moderate' need and still less on those whose need the assessors considered to be 'slight'. Indeed, in the special group those with considerable need had almost twice as much help in relation to all three activities – visits, contact with other agencies and practical help – as those with slight need; those whose

TABLE V. 11

AVERAGE NUMBER OF VISITS, CONTACTS WITH OTHER AGENCIES AND ITEMS OF PRACTICAL HELP, COMPARED WITH THE ASSESSORS' JUDGEMENTS OF 'INDICATIONS FOR SOCIAL WORK'.

'Indications for social work'	Average no. of visits		Average no. of agencies contacted		Average no. of items of practical help	
	Special group (N=110)	Comparison group (N=104)	Special group (N=110)	Comparison group (N=104)	Special group (N=110)	Comparison group (N=104)
Considerable	20·9	10·7	6·3	3·5	6·1	2·2
Moderate	14·7	6·9	4·4	2·2	3·8	1·8
Slight/none	10·6	6·2	3·7	1·9	2·9	1·5
No evidence (1 case only)	15·0	—	7·0	—	4·0	—

needs were rated as 'moderate' fall neatly in the middle. The trend is not as steep in the comparison group.

This is of considerable interest, since we know (Table V. 5) that the social workers in the comparison group did not differentiate categories of need as clearly as the social workers in the special group; the former included nearly two-thirds of their cases in the 'moderate' need category. It looks as though their social work activities were correspondingly less differentiated. These are important observations from which we draw three conclusions:

First of all: the finding that the project social workers worked more differentially indicates something about the quality of their work and their decision making which cannot merely be explained by the fact that they had more time at their disposal. This will be discussed in more detail in the concluding chapter.

Secondly: even on one visit in which much background material had to be gathered an experienced social worker could apparently make a useful assessment of the indications for social work which stood the test of events and of the actual social work carried out by people who were completely unaware of this independent assessment.

Thirdly: the validity of this judgement also indicates that it would be quite feasible to assign after one initial assessment the care for different kinds of cases to workers with different degrees of training and experience.

Outcome as Seen by the Social Workers

Although the workers in the special group were able to make a more intensive and differentiated effort to help their clients, yet their judgements about outcome were more cautious than that of their colleagues. They thought that just over half (55 per cent) were 'better' in relation to their initial problems while the workers in the comparison group thought that 63 per cent had improved. The project social workers felt that 15 per cent were worse off, whereas the social workers in the comparison group thought that only 8 per cent had deteriorated.

The social workers were asked to give evidence for their judgements. In the majority of cases the improvement claimed consisted in a reduction of practical needs; in a smaller proportion of cases they claimed that attitudes had changed for the better. The social workers very rarely suggested that their clients were better off in all respects, that is to say in relation to their physical capacity, their situation and their psychological adjustment.

Finally we asked the social workers what problems still remained after ten months of social work (Table V. 12). Comparing the problems present at the end of the social work period with the initial problems it is again noticeable how realistic the social workers in both groups were.

TABLE V. 12

PROBLEMS SEEN BY SOCIAL WORKERS AT BEGINNING AND END OF
THE EXPERIMENT
(Percentage distributions)

Type of problem	Special group (N=110)		Comparison group (N=104)	
	Beginning	End	Beginning	End
Physical disability	92	91	86	80
Housing	29	22	33	21
Financial difficulties	11	9	3	2
Poor home conditions/Inability to cope	5	3	6	3
Burden on family	10	6	5	5
Social isolation/Loneliness	45	20	47	37
Difficulty in personal relations	20	12	9	6
Mental and emotional disorder worries and anxieties }	40	31	24	17
Miscellaneous	6	2	4	1

They saw a decrease in problems in some respects but felt that many difficulties still remained. Clearly physical disability among this very elderly group had hardly changed at all. It is interesting that the social workers in the special group saw a much greater reduction in problems of isolation and loneliness than the workers in the comparison group. This might have sprung from their efforts to relieve depression, to introduce voluntary visitors, to encourage their clients to join clubs, to go on holidays and from their own frequent contact with them. The social workers in the comparison group knew that they had not been able to visit as much as they wished; they had found few voluntary visitors and thus did not feel that they had relieved much loneliness or isolation. The picture in relation to mental and emotional disorder and other kinds of anxieties shows little change which is probably a realistic estimate. Similarly both groups of workers still thought that about a fifth of their clients had housing problems.

In Summary
A brief look at the social-work effort extending over ten months in both groups showed that in every respect the social workers in the special group put in about double the amount of work as was possible for the workers in the comparison group. The project social workers' perception of the old person's needs and of their casework role differed considerably from that of their colleagues in the comparison group. They saw more problems, their prescriptions contained more emphasis on casework and work with relatives. They worked much more closely with medical agencies, with many different voluntary agencies and with volunteers; they made greater efforts to enrich their clients' lives by introducing them to clubs, by encouraging holidays and outings and by drawing in volunteers. In their casework they encouraged more ventilation of feelings, discussion of past and present relationships and they used their clarifying role more, both with clients and relatives, and with social agencies. They worked more selectively according to people's needs, giving twice as much help to those judged by the independent assessors to be in considerable need of social work as to those with minimal needs. At the same time their judgements on outcome were a little more cautious than those of the social workers in the comparison group.

References
Cavan, R. S. (1962): *Self and Role in Adjustment During Old Age*, in: Rose, A. (editor), *Human Behaviour and Social Processes*, Routledge, pp. 526–36.
Cumming, E. and Henry, W. E. (1961): *Growing Old. Process of Disengagement*, New York, Basic Books.
Jefferys, M. (1965): *An Anatomy of Social Welfare Services*, Michael Joseph.

6

THE E   ECTS OF SOCIAL WORK

We have seen that the special group received significantly more social work, both practical and supportive, directly through face-to-face contacts and indirectly through contacts with other agencies than the comparison group. The crucial question we wish to explore in this chapter is: were the effects of these intensive efforts made by the trained social workers different from the results achieved by the social workers who carried larger caseloads, and who did not have the benefit of professional social work training?

After $10\frac{1}{2}$ months, the social work and the medical assessors interviewed all the survivors in the sample using the same questionnaire as on the first occasion, but they did not see their first interview schedule before their visits. Some questions were added to elicit the old people's feelings and attitudes about the help they had received. As the study was geared to social work with the elderly living in the community the final comparisons were restricted to those living in their own homes. The circumstances of the clients who were reinterviewed in hospital or in residential homes were discussed in Chapter IV.

Reassessment
The assessors had a separate office in the administrative block of the welfare department, and had only minimal contact with the social workers in either group and never discussed any cases with them. They were of course unaware which subjects had been allocated to the special or comparison group. Nor did they know what kind of social work had taken place in the intervening period. However, by the end of the interview the name of the social worker concerned had been mentioned by 64 per cent of the clients in the special group, and by 32 per cent of those in the comparison group. The questions most likely to reveal the identity of the social worker, those which concerned the old people's

contacts with social workers and their satisfaction with the services, were deliberately asked at the end of the interview. It is therefore reasonable to assume that where the clients did mention their social worker's name the assessors did not know until the end of the interview to which group the welfare client belonged and that any possible bias was reduced to a minimum. It is of course striking that names were mentioned twice as often in the special as in the comparison group. This is almost certainly related to two factors; first, the social workers in the special group had been in much more frequent contact with their clients than the other social workers; secondly, in over half of the cases in the comparison group more than one social worker had visited the old person.

In accordance with the criteria of outcome discussed in Chapter II, we shall try to assess differential success and failure in four areas:

1. *environmental changes* in relation to housing, finance and services received;
2. *changes in functioning* as expressed in personal capacity, state of health, diet, general activities and social contacts;
3. *changes in subjective attitudes* and feelings expressed by the clients about themselves and the world around them;
4. *changes in the social work assessors' judgements* about the extent and nature of practical needs, the degree and type of 'problems' experienced, and the clients' contentment.

Changes can be assessed in three different ways.

I One can look at the difference in *outcome between the groups* and compare the state of the clients in the special group with that of the clients in the comparison group at the end of the experiment. For example by the end of the experiment 40 per cent of the clients in the special and 27 per cent of the clients in the comparison group were going to clubs.

II One can look at the *movement within each group between first and second assessments*, comparing the clients' state at the end of the experiment with their state at the beginning. For example 25 per cent of the clients in the special group reported that they were attending clubs when first assessed and 40 per cent at the second assessment. Twenty-nine per cent of the clients in the comparison group said that they were attending clubs on first assessment and 27 per cent on second assessment.

III One can look at the *difference in movement between the two groups*. For example 15 per cent of the clients in the special group joined a club during the experiment and none in the comparison group.

In the subsequent analysis of the material we shall pay attention to these three measures of which movements within and between the groups are probably the most important.

Clearly in some of these areas social work intervention is likely to have more effect than in others. For instance, given the present housing situation in London, changes in housing will rarely be achieved within 10 months; or again, among such an elderly and incapacitated population one would not expect a general improvement in health. We recognized these constraints in the formulation of our hypotheses referred to on p. 41. On the whole, as will be shown, the findings confirm our expectations as to where changes were likely to occur.[1]

Environmental Changes
Housing and Finance. Housing amenities hardly changed in either group and what changes there were – a few more inside lavatories and fixed baths – were the results of rehousing. Thirteen old people had moved house, 6 in the special and 7 in the comparison group. In the limited time available in one interview it was not possible to determine accurately changes in other amenities such as the fixing of hand rails and fire guards or the more convenient placing of a gas meter, and so on. Although the social workers put much effort into this kind of work, (Table V. 8, p. 115) the only measurable indication of outcome in this sphere was some improvement in the means of heating the bedroom. Ten per cent more of the old people in the special group and 5 per cent more in the comparison group had some means of heating their bed-rooms at the second assessment. Similarly, the financial situation was difficult to ascertain accurately. The number in receipt of supplementary benefits remained practically the same in both groups. There is a suggestion that the financial situation of the special group improved.

[1] A note on the methods of analysis will be found in Appendix 2. The findings discussed in this chapter relate to straight comparisons between answers to individual questions. As will be seen from the appendix a component analysis was also carried out from which eleven factors emerged.

The proportion of clients who found difficulty in meeting expenses decreased from 45 per cent to 40 per cent in the special group, but increased from 34 per cent to 45 per cent in the comparison group. This possibly reflects the efforts of the social workers in the special group to obtain increases in supplementary allowances or discretionary grants in suitable cases (see Chapter V, p. 120 and also Table V. 8).

Services Received. In Chapter III we considered the services and the kind of help this sample of old people appeared to need in addition to domiciliary services they were already receiving. We have also seen how active the social workers had been in both groups, and particularly in the special group in arranging practical help for their clients. The expectations therefore are that significantly more clients will report receiving various kinds of social services and social work help on the second visit than did on the first interview. Table VI. 1 which enumerates some of the services received in each group at first and second assessment does not confirm these expectations in every respect.

TABLE VI. 1

WELFARE CLIENTS' REPORTS OF SERVICES RECEIVED
(Percentage distributions)

Type of service	Special group (N=110)		Comparison group (N=104)	
	1st Ass.	*2nd Ass.*	*1st Ass.*	*2nd Ass.*
Home help	48	56	55	58
Meals on Wheels	27	29	31	36
Chiropody	45	54	42	51
District Nurse	5	10	12	8
Clubs	25	40	29	27
Holiday (within the last year)	26	45	32	34
Voluntary visitor	24	24	22	19

It may seem disappointing at first sight that there was such a small increase in the delivery of meals-on-wheels and the provision of home helps in both groups; but one has to remember that about half of the old people already had home helps at the first assessment and just over a quarter were receiving meals-on-wheels.

On their first visits the social work assessors considered that an additional 10 per cent in both groups needed home helps and 7 per cent meals-on-wheels. Thus the small increase almost achieved this 'need' target, for on the second visit the social work assessors considered that no one in the special group and 5 per cent in the comparison group needed additional meals-on-wheels and only 2 per cent in the special and 4 per cent in the comparison group additional home help (see Table VI. 7 p. 146). Nine per cent more of the clients in both groups reported that they were receiving chiropody services. The degree of improvement noted in relation to foot problems by the medical assessor is very similar. The proportion of old people found to have 'no foot problems' on the second medical assessment increased by 9 per cent in the special group (from 13 per cent to 22 per cent) and by 6 per cent in the comparison group (from 22 per cent to 28 per cent). Once more one can detect hardly any differences in outcome between the two groups. This was not to be expected since the social work effort concerned with chiropody was roughly the same in both groups (see Table V. 8 p. 115).

In contrast, club and day centre attendances had increased significantly in the special group from 25 per cent on the first visit to 40 per cent on the second, but they had remained virtually the same in the comparison group – 29 per cent on the first and 27 per cent on the second assessment (Table VI. 1). The difference in outcome *between* the two groups is not quite significant statistically (40 per cent attending clubs in the special group and 27 per cent in the comparison group), because the special group started with somewhat lower attendances; but the difference in movement between the two groups is significant (Table 6, Appendix 1). A 40 per cent attendance at club and day centres in the special group seems a remarkable achievement, considering that nearly half the clientele were over eighty years of age. It seems then that the great effort which the project social workers invested in encouraging people to try clubs and day centres and motivating them by taking them along personally and introducing them to those in charge had visible results. Close inspection and comparison of the social work claims in Table V. 8, p. 115 with the results shown in Table VI. 1 of this chapter reveals discrepancies. The social workers claim to have achieved club or day centre attendances for 35 per cent of their clients, but the increase reported by the old people themselves was only 15 per cent. Scrutiny of the case records showed that in a number of cases the social workers had arranged additional club attendances and in a few instances the old person had lapsed just before the final assessment. In only 3 cases (1 in the special and 2 in the comparison group) were the claims of the social workers not substantiated.

The other significant change which occurred in the special and not in the comparison group was the increase in the number of old people who said that they had a holiday in the previous year. This proportion rose from 26 per cent to 45 per cent in the special group and remained virtually the same in the comparison group (Table VI. 1). This difference in movement between the two groups was significant although the difference in outcome was not; 45 per cent having had a holiday in the special group compared with 34 per cent in the comparison group. The most surprising feature of Table VI. 1 is the apparent lack of increase in voluntary visiting in both groups, which is in great contrast to the claims of the social workers in the special groups who reported that they had achieved voluntary visiting and other voluntary help in 32 per cent of the cases. There are various explanations for this. We have evidence that some clients who said that they had no voluntary visits were in fact being visited by a volunteer; in other cases the voluntary visits were erratic or unsuccessful (as described in the previous chapter), either because the old person did not take to a young schoolgirl coming in about five o'clock or the youngster herself did not see the point of 'just visiting'. In addition the old people had great difficulty in identifying the different people who were calling on them or in understanding the 'labels' attached to different kinds of helpers about whom the assessors asked them in the interview. The clients may well have had a voluntary visitor in mind when replying to the question, 'Has a welfare officer called on you?'. This was answered in the affirmative by 94 per cent of clients in the special and 77 per cent in the comparison group – a statistically highly significant difference. Be that as it may, it seems that one of the major efforts in this project, namely to draw in volunteers could not be reliably measured in terms of self reports by the old people in an interview.

Physical and Social Functioning of the Old People.
We now want to examine whether social work had any effect on the physical and social functioning of the clients, that is to say on their incapacity to look after themselves, as measured by the incapacity score and the functional movement rating; on the state of their health, on their nutritional state as measured by their protein intake; on the extent

and nature of their activities as measured by the activity score and lastly on the extent of their social contacts.

Capacity and Health. No one would expect a group of aged and incapacitated welfare clients to improve significantly in their ability to walk, negotiate stairs or cut their toe-nails. But one of our hypotheses was that the old people in the special group would show less deterioration on scores for self-care and household capacity than the comparison group (Chapter II, p. 41). This is borne out not by the assessments made on the second visit. In the special group the proportion of those with no or slight incapacity had increased a little and the proportion

TABLE VI. 2

CAPACITY AND HEALTH
(Percentage distributions)

	Special group (N=110)		Comparison group (N=104)	
	1st Ass.	*2nd Ass.*	*1st Ass.*	*2nd Ass.*
Personal incapacity				
None or slight	23	30	27	26
Fair	37	30	26	30
Moderate	20	20	21	21
Severe	20	20	26	23
	(N=101*)		(N=96*)	
Functional movement				
Good	35	36	39	31
Fair	48	49	44	56
Poor	16	16	17	11
No evidence	2	0	0	1
Breathlessness				
None	66	52	70	62
Breathless walking across room	30	38	23	29
Breathless sitting and talking	3	7	4	4
Breathless sitting at rest	1	2	3	5
No evidence	0	1	0	0
Medical condition				
No or slight illness	41	29	35	28
Stabilized medical condition	43	50	51	43
Serious illness threatening life	17	21	14	29

* The medical assessor carried out assessments and reassessments on 101 clients in the special and 96 clients in the comparison group.

with a 'fair' amount of incapacity to begin with decreased. The number of those whose incapacity was moderate and severe remained the same. In the comparison group the differences between the first and second assessments were even smaller.

It is somewhat surprising that neither group reported much deterioration in their capacity to manage daily tasks and that their functional movement, as observed by the medical assessor, had not decreased, especially, as their general health had declined (Table VI. 2). For instance, 29 per cent of the special group were rated as having no, or very slight illness at the end compared with 41 per cent at the start, whilst in the comparison group this drop was not quite so great, 35 per cent having the highest rating on health at the beginning and 28 per cent at the end. There was also evidence of increased breathlessness in both groups and slight deterioration in their haemoglobin measure.

Serious illness considered by the physician to threaten life, and deaths affected the two groups somewhat differently. We proposed the hypothesis that more old people in the special group would survive than in the comparison group (Chapter II, p. 41). Of the 48 welfare clients who died, 21 were in the special and 27 in the comparison group. Although the trend is in the direction of our hypothesis this difference is, of course, by no means statistically significant. However, any possible effect may have been masked because of more adverse circumstances in the special group which, though small, persist in every sphere (Table IV. 5, p. 94): more in the special group were severely ill (17 per cent compared with 14 per cent), more had psychiatric conditions (13 per cent compared with 11 per cent), more had 4 or more practical needs (23 per cent with 15 per cent), more were severely depressed (24 per cent compared with 20 per cent), and were found to have pronounced personal problems (17 per cent compared with 12 per cent); the comparison group also had more contact with their children and had received more help from them, than the special group. The only important factor favouring the special group and leading one to expect fewer deaths is that they were somewhat younger: initially 60 per cent were under eighty compared with 55 per cent in the comparison group. This factor may well have been the decisive one accounting for fewer deaths in the special group, but it is possible that the extensive services provided, the support given and the close collaboration with medical agencies contributed to this outcome. This suggestion finds an echo if we look at those who, in the opinion of the medical assessor, had a serious medical condition threatening life. The table shows that on his first assessment more people were in this category in the special group – 17 per cent compared with 14 per cent in the comparison group. On the second assessment there were fewer – 21 per cent in the special group and 29 per cent in the comparison group. In other words only 4 people had been added to the ranks of the seriously ill during the 10 months in the special group, but there were 15 more seriously ill clients in the comparison group; and while 80 clients did not deteriorate to the seriously ill category in the special group, this only applied to 68 old people in the comparison group. This difference in movement is statistically significant (Table 6, Appendix 1) and cannot be explained by the possibility of more hospital admissions in the special group, since equal proportions from both groups were in hospital on second assessment.

There was no evidence in either group of any improvement in two important areas of functioning – sight and hearing. Despite the ophthalmic assessments arranged by some of the social workers there was only minimal improvement in the ability of the old people to read lettering of newsprint size at the end of the period. In the comparison group the proportion able to do so declined slightly. Similarly, although ears had been syringed and wax removed in some cases, the proportion of old people with impaired ability to hear the spoken voice increased at the second assessment. Encouragingly, some old people who were only slightly deaf to start with improved in hearing in both groups by the end of the experiment. Removal of wax may have enabled them to enjoy their social contacts better. Similarly, the clients in both groups were still afflicted by as many minor discomforts and disabilities on their second as on their first medical assessment (Table VI. 3). Since they were in poorer health and no better off with respect to their special senses or their ability to move about, this was probably to be expected. The symptoms especially inquired for were giddiness, poor appetite, inability to masticate adequately, urinary symptoms, constipation, poor sleep, poor eyesight, poor hearing and foot discomforts. There was a trend for clients in both the special and the comparison groups to report the presence of a greater number of components of this 'misery syndrome' on the second occasion (Table VI. 3). Interestingly, once again, in the worst group, that is to say those experiencing five or more complaints, the proportion of clients in the special group remained virtually the same, while there was an increase

TABLE VI. 3

MINOR DISCOMFORTS AND DISABILITIES
(Percentage distributions)

Number of Complaints	Special group (N=101*)		Comparison group (N=96*)	
	1st Ass.	2nd Ass.	1st Ass.	2nd Ass.
0	6	7	8	8
1 – 2	41	32	35	33
3 – 4	29	38	38	32
5 or more	23	22	16	22
No evidence	1	1	3	5
Average no. of complaints	2·9	3·1	2·7	2·9

* See footnote Table VI, 2.

of 6 per cent in the comparison group. This increase in the miseries of old age represents the inexorable deterioration in bodily health, but one also wonders whether the social workers had failed to spot these troubles and to bring in medical aid for those discomforts which were remediable. These problems will be discussed further in the final chapter.

Diet. We mentioned earlier that the social workers in both groups were notified of those clients whose diet scores indicated a very low protein intake. We did this because we wanted to explore whether social workers could exert any influence on their elderly clients' nutrition. The social workers in the special group paid a great deal of attention to improving the diet of those who were notified to them as possibly undernourished, particularly during the first months, when they had as yet a comparatively small caseload. Table VI. 4 shows a small but distinct improvement among those with low protein diets in the special group. The proportion of these clients decreased from 21 per cent to 14 per cent at the second assessment while the proportion of the poorly nourished remained virtually the same in the comparison group. Furthermore, we know from inspection of cases that this improvement in the special group is almost entirely accounted for by clients who came into the study early on, when the social workers were able to pay very special attention to their diet. It looks as though social workers can contribute to the improvement of old people's diet if they are alerted to this need and give it special attention.

TABLE VI. 4

DIET

(Percentage distributions)

Quantity of protein	Special group (N=110)		Comparison group (N=104)	
	1st Ass.	*2nd Ass.*	*1st Ass.*	*2nd Ass.*
Low	21	14	23	22
Medium	46	45	39	37
High	29	36	36	38
No evidence	4	5	2	4

Activities. It will be recalled that we constructed an activity score which seeks to discriminate between those old people who initiate physical or mental activity (for example shopping, reading, seeing other people at home or elsewhere) and those who live a passive life (for instance sitting and thinking, sleeping, watching people go by in the street, and so on). In one of our hypotheses we postulated that more people in the special than in the comparison group would increase their interests and activities (Chapter II, p. 41). This hypothesis has stood the test. Whereas the groups differed little on the initial assessment, the final assessment showed a significant difference between the two groups – a greater proportion (50 per cent) of the clients in the special group scoring above average than in the comparison group (34 per cent) (Table VI. 5). This result is clearly related to the encouragement the old people in the special group received to join clubs and day centres and to go there more often and to take an interest in 'real life' rather than merely in reminiscences and fantasies. We also know (see Table V. 8, p. 115) that the social workers in the special group arranged many more outings for the old people than the social workers in the comparison group and that the clients in the special group had had more holidays. This increase in activity is remarkable, considering how old and incapacitated these elderly welfare clients were, that they had deteriorated in health and that they suffered more inconvenience from minor symptoms.

Social Contacts. It is generally assumed that social work, both in the form of practical support and as a therapeutic relationship, can enable people to function better socially and to feel more at ease in their personal relationships. We thus advanced the hypothesis that more old

TABLE VI. 5

SOCIAL FUNCTIONING
(Percentage distributions)

	Special group		Comparison group	
	1st Ass.	2nd Ass.	1st Ass.	2nd Ass.
Activity score	(N=110)		(N=104)	
Low	21	15	22	16
Medium	36	35	40	49
High	30	35	27	29
Very high	13	15	9	5
No evidence	0	0	2	1
Number of contacts with children in past 7 days	(N=74*)		(N=62*)	
None	32	32	15	16
1 − 3	24	19	22	24
4 − 9	18	26	32	32
10 or more	26	23	31	26
No evidence	0	0	0	2
Number of people seen yesterday	(N=110)		(N=104)	
0	6	7	5	6
1	2	14	17	17
2	25	24	33	32
3	25	20	18	20
4+	24	34	26	24
No evidence	0	2	1	1

* Only applies to those with children.

people in the special than in the comparison group would improve their social contacts with family, neighbours and friends. That this is not borne out by the findings is shown in Table VI. 5. It should be noted, however, that the information only relates to the amount and not to the quality of the contacts. Little change appears to have occurred between the first and second assessments in relation to contacts with children. It is perhaps particularly disappointing that the percentage of those not seeing any of their children in the week preceding the interview (32 per cent and 15 per cent respectively in the special and comparison groups) had remained the same. On going further into this, we found that practically all these cases related to children who lived more than half an hour's journey away from their parents. Still, half an hour or more is not a long journey these days. It looks as if both sets of social workers did not succeed, or perhaps did not think it relevant to stimulate more contact between the old people and children who did not live in the immediate vicinity. There is a suggestion that children in the special group were helping their parents more at the end of the experiment – a 9 per cent increase – while in the comparison group they seemed to help considerably less – a 16 per cent decrease. This may be an indication of improvement in the quality rather than in the quantity of the relationships. Examples from the social work described in the last chapter will come to mind (p. 111). The number of people the clients had seen on the day preceding the interview also did not change substantially in either group, though it will be noted that 10 per cent of the clients in the special group saw 4 or more people on their second assessment while the comparison group did not move in this respect. Nor could differences be detected either within or between the two groups in relation to contacts with friends or neighbours. Perhaps such a widening of contacts cannot reasonably be expected in such an aged group, although efforts by the local community itself and neighbourhood meeting facilities could possibly encompass even some very old and incapacitated people.

Subjective Attitudes
Although we expected few if any changes in outcome in relation to the old people's physical environment, and only modest improvements in their functioning we hoped that any practical and psychological support the social workers were able to give their welfare clients would contribute to a greater sense of well-being and satisfaction with life.

We thus stated as one of our hypotheses that more old people in the special than in the comparison group would show positive changes in their attitudes to their present situation as measured by the attitude rating score (Chapter II, p. 41). There are a number of indications that this has happened (Table VI. 6).

For instance, in their answer to the question 'What do you feel about your life at the moment?' a significantly greater proportion of the clients in the special group said they were 'satisfied' on the second assessment than on the first (71 per cent compared with 58 per cent) and fewer felt dissatisfied, a drop from 19 per cent to 6 per cent. There was

TABLE VI. 6

SUBJECTIVE ATTITUDES
(Percentage distributions)

Attitude	Special group (N=110)		Comparison group (N=104)	
	1st Ass.	2nd Ass.	1st Ass.	2nd Ass.
Satisfaction with life at the moment				
Satisfied	58	71	63	70
Mixed feelings	21	19	19	14
Dissatisfied	19	6	15	13
No evidence	2	4	2	3
Attitude to outside world				
Good	25	29	26	26
Fair	34	36	37	26
Poor	34	17	32	32
No evidence	6	17	6	16
Client's evaluation of health				
Good	65	78	64	74
Fair	27	15	28	18
Poor	7	6	7	6
No evidence	1	2	1	2
Loneliness				
Never lonely	65	62	62	62
Sometimes lonely	21	26	28	24
Often lonely	14	9	10	13
No evidence	0	3	1	1
Worry				
No worries	35	49	46	52
Worried about one thing	44	35	45	35
Worried about more than one thing	18	11	7	10
No evidence	4	5	2	4
Depression	(N=101)*		(N=96)*	
Very little depression	24	45	28	35
Some depression	50	30	52	46
Serious depression	24	24	20	16
No evidence	3	2	0	3

* See footnote Table VI. 2

also a small increase in satisfaction in the comparison group (from 63 per cent to 70 per cent), but the proportion of those dissatisfied hardly changed at all. Once more, although the difference between first and second assessment was significant *within* the special group it did not lead to a significant difference in outcome *between* the two groups, that is to say at the end of the experiment 71 per cent in the special group and 70 per cent in the comparison group said that they felt satisfied with life at the moment. The reason for this may be that the special group started from a somewhat worse position, since the difference in move-ment between the 2 groups was statistically significant. On the other hand, the change that occurred in attitudes to the outside world did lead to a significant difference in outcome *between* the groups. A number of statements were read to the old people and after each they were asked whether they agreed, disagreed or felt neutral. Each person was given a score based on the replies. In the special group, 17 per cent expressed negative attitudes on the second occasion, compared with 32 per cent in the comparison group (Table VI. 6). Unfortunately, this measure loses some of its value, as on the second occasion 36 people were unable to concentrate sufficiently well to be scored, but since the failures were evenly distributed between the two groups (17 per cent and 16 per cent) some importance can be attached to the differences that emerged among the rest.

This growth of positive feelings is also noticeable in the replies to questions about worry and depression.

Clients, particularly those in the special group, expressed fewer worries at their second assessment. Those who said that they had no worries increased by 14 per cent in the special group and by 6 per cent in the comparison group. Once more, this greater movement within the special group is not reflected in differences in outcome (Table VI. 6).

It may be recalled that a depression score was derived from three answers concerned with depression: 'Do you get depressed nowadays?', 'How often do you feel depressed?', and 'How long does the depression last?'. Table VI. 6 shows that the proportion of those least depressed had increased significantly in the special group (from 24 per cent to 45 per cent), while in the comparison group the improvement was much smaller (from 28 per cent to 35 per cent). This difference in movement between the groups also proved to be significant (Table 6, Appendix 1). It should be noted that among the most depressed no change occurred in the special group, but there was a slight decrease of very depressed people in the comparison group. A greater sense of well-being and satisfaction could also be observed in feelings related to situations which objectively had not improved at all. On the whole the clients' health had deteriorated, yet on the second visit more people in both groups considered their health to be good (either in a qualified or unqualified way) and this trend was a little more marked in the special than in the comparison group. Similarly, although there had been so little objective improvement in their housing conditions, yet, 83 per cent of the special group expressed satisfaction (either qualified or unqualified) with their housing on the second assessment compared with 71 per cent on the first occasion, while satisfaction had lessened by two cases in the comparison group. And those dissatisfied had decreased by 13 per cent in the special group while there was no change in the comparison group.

Interestingly, feelings of loneliness hardly changed at all in either group (Table VI.6); nearly two-thirds maintained, as they did on the assessors' first visit that they were *never* lonely. On the face of it, it seems unlikely that nearly two-thirds of these elderly, incapacitated people, most of whom lived alone, should never feel lonely. This may denote the old people's resignation and acceptance of their way of life as 'natural' for old age. It is also possible that in our age which places such a high premium on 'other-directedness' (Rieseman, 1961) and so much emphasis on skill in relationships, people may feel shame in admitting loneliness.

The general increase in contentment and in more positive attitudes to the world around them in the special group, and to a much lesser extent in the comparison group, may well be related to the support, both practical and psychological, provided by the social workers and to the enriching experiences in clubs, on holidays and on outings.

The Needs and Problems of Clients as Judged by the Assessors
Lastly, the social work assessors, who were of course unaware of the kind of help the welfare clients received in the intervening period, used their social work knowledge and insight to assess the old people's needs. These needs were either expressed by the clients themselves or observed by the assessor.

Inspection of Table VI. 7 shows that the assessors found far fewer unmet practical needs on their second visits. This reduction is statistically highly significant in both groups. On the first round nearly every-

TABLE VI. 7

ASSESSORS' JUDGEMENTS OF PRESENCE OF PRACTICAL NEEDS
(Percentage distributions)

	Special group (N=110)		Comparison group (N=104)	
	1st Ass.	2nd Ass.	1st Ass.	2nd Ass.
Number of practical needs 0	7	41	10	28
1	25	34	25	34
2	23	15	27	18
3	23	8	23	7
4	12	2	10	10
5+	10	0	5	3
Average number of practical needs	2·4	0·9	2·1	1·5
Types of need				
Housing				
Rehousing	14	11	11	11
Sheltered housing	5	11	13	10
Permanent residential care	1	1	2	2
Domiciliary services				
Home help	10	2	10	4
Meals on Wheels	7	0	7	5
Adaptations	8	3	4	1
Aids (for handicapped)	4	1	8	5
'Good Neighbour' service	5	0	4	1
Library	6	1	5	3
Help with garden	1	1	1	3
House repairs and redecoration	9	5	3	14
Health services				
Chiropody	25	15	23	19
Medical attention	17	4	10	10
District Nurse/Bathing Service	6	2	4	2
Community facilities				
Club/day centre	27	5	28	9
Holiday	18	4	25	15
Outings	4	2	6	4
Material aid				
Financial help	9	2	5	5
Supply of clothes, bed linen, furniture	11	5	3	3
Loan of TV	10	4	8	5
Loan of wireless	5	3	4	3
Visiting services				
Visiting of volunteer	28	6	20	7
Advice and information	2	4	6	12
Miscellaneous	2	4	1	3

body was judged to have some practical needs, but on the second assessment two fifths of the special group (41 per cent) and just over a quarter in the comparison group (28 per cent) were thought to have no outstanding practical needs. At the other extreme 22 per cent of the clients in the special group appeared to have 4 or more needs on the first visit, and this proportion was reduced to 2 per cent on the second assessment; in the comparison group the corresponding reduction was only very small, from 15 per cent to 13 per cent. In other words, while the social work assessors discovered significantly fewer practical needs after 10 months' social work in both groups, this reduction was even greater in the special group, so that there is also a statistically significant difference in outcome *between* the groups on the second assessment. The average need reduction (i.e. the number of needs on first assessment minus those on the second assessment) was 1·5 for the special group and 0·6 for the comparison group. This outcome closely matches the reported input of practical help, the workers in the special group reporting on average over twice as much practical help achieved (3·9 items of service per person) as the workers in the comparison group (1·8 items of service per person).

This congruence between input and outcome is also apparent if we examine the changes in individual needs. It does not come as a surprise that needs with respect to housing had hardly altered in either group, in fact in the assessors' opinion the need for sheltered housing had increased in the special group. The social workers in both groups, as well as the assessors, estimated that around one fifth of the clients were in need of rehousing at the end of the experiment (compare Table V. 11). The other substantial remaining need was for chiropody. Fifteen per cent of the clients in the special and 19 per cent in the comparison group still appeared to be in need of this service, although there had been some reduction in the number requiring footcare, particularly in the special group – 10 per cent. These findings again fit well with the social workers' account of their work; they reported that in the special group they had arranged chiropody for 16 per cent of the clients and in the comparison group for 13 per cent of cases. But the initial social assessment and the medical examination revealed that at least a quarter of the old people needed attention for their feet. So there was room for an ever greater effort on the part of the social workers.

We have already noted the significant increase in the number of welfare clients in the special group, who told the assessors that they were attending clubs and day centres and had a holiday during the preceding year. This clearly led to a greatly reduced need in these directions. A more complex phenomenon is the considerably reduced need for voluntary visiting, as seen by the social work assessors. On the face of it this could reflect the project social workers' great drive in this sphere, but (as Table VI. 1 showed) the old people themselves reported no increase in voluntary visitors. We suggested that the clients may have been unable to distinguish clearly between the various types of visitors. There is another possible explanation for the discrepancy between the clients' and the assessors' judgements. The assessors may have felt that the clients were receiving other forms of care and that they were somewhat more active and in touch with other people, for instance in clubs and, therefore, no longer in need of the help and companionship of volunteers. Lastly, we cannot exclude the possibility that the assessors had in fact altered their criteria without realizing it, especially as the 'young volunteers' were not always well received by the elderly.

Another interesting finding in Table VI. 7 is that in the assessors' estimate the need for medical attention had decreased dramatically in the special group, from 17 per cent to 4 per cent, while it had stayed the same at 10 per cent in the comparison group. This may well reflect the project social workers' much greater contact with general practitioners and other medical agencies on behalf of their clients.

There is also an indication that the project social workers' efforts in relation to their clients' financial situation was perceived by the assessors.

A puzzling result shown in Table VI.7 is the apparent increase in the need for home repairs and decoration in the comparison group. This need had decreased in the special group where the social workers said that they had helped in 8 cases. Does this apparent deterioration of the physical surroundings reflect the local authority social workers' time pressures which force them to concentrate on the clients' immediate personal needs and comforts? In this case it seems unlikely that the assessors had changed their standards, as their judgements fit in with the special group workers' reported efforts.

The assessors also attempted to sum up their impressions about the nature of the old persons' difficulties and the degree of their contentment, taking account of everything they had absorbed during their interviews with the clients (Table VI. 8). These more clinical and holistic judgements mirror substantially what has already become apparent from the clients' own responses to questions.

TABLE VI. 8

ASSESSORS' CLINICAL JUDGEMENTS
(Percentage distributions)

Type of problem	Special group (N=110)		Comparison group (N=104)	
	1st Ass.	2nd Ass.	1st Ass.	2nd Ass.
Environmental difficulties				
Pronounced	12	5	10	9
Moderate	30	25	33	26
Slight	51	56	50	57
None	7	14	8	9
Interpersonal difficulties				
Pronounced	7	5	5	4
Moderate	9	6	7	5
Slight	20	17	19	21
None	62	66	59	63
No evidence	2	5	11	8
Personal problems				
Pronounced	17	9	12	16
Moderate	41	26	44	29
Slight	28	46	32	42
None	14	19	12	12
Contentment				
Contented	12	19	14	17
Fairly contented	45	49	38	51
Neither contented nor discontented	17	17	20	16
Discontented	17	11	13	10
Openly unhappy	8	2	13	6
No evidence	1	2	1	0

While their environmental difficulties (which included housing, finance and the provision of services) had only moderately improved in the special group and hardly at all in the comparison group, the clients' personal problems had been reduced significantly in the special group, but considerably less in the comparison group. The proportion of clients who were judged to have pronounced personal problems decreased by 8 per cent in the special group and increased by 4 per cent in the comparison group; while the proportion of those with slight or no problems increased by 23 per cent in the special group and by 10 per cent in the comparison group.

The social work assessors' judgements of the clients' contentment differed in some respects from the clients' own reports about their satisfaction with life at the moment. The assessors attributed greater improvement in contentment to the comparison group (16 per cent) than to the special group (11 per cent), while of the old people themselves fewer reported an increase in their feelings of satisfaction in the comparison group (7 per cent) than in the special group (13 per cent) (see Table VI. 6). At the other end of the scale the assessors' judgements suggest that discontentment and unhappiness had decreased in a similar fashion in both groups. Yet the old people's answers indicate a considerable decrease in the numbers dissatisfied in the special group, and hardly any change in the comparison group (Table VI. 6). Thus the assessors attributed more improvement to the comparison group than the reports of the clients themselves indicate. This suggests that the assessors were not biased in favour of the special group although the names of the social workers had been mentioned by the end of the interview in about two-thirds of the special group cases.

In Summary
Significant Differences in Outcome Between Special and Comparison Groups. Comparing the effect of social work in the special and comparison groups on a large number of variables we found few statistically significant differences in outcome between the groups. They were as follows: more clients in the special group reported contacts with a social worker, they also reported greater activity, revealed more positive attitudes to the outside world and reported less depression than the clients in the comparison group. The assessors reported more reduction in practical needs in the special than in the comparison group. In other respects the outcomes in the two groups were not significantly different despite the very much greater and different efforts by the social workers in the special group.

Significant Changes Within the Two Groups. We also observed a number of statistically significant differences between the first and second assessment, all but one within the special group which were always in the direction of improvement. Significantly more old people in the special group were attending clubs and day centres, had had a holiday, felt satisfied with life at the moment, had a more positive attitude to the world around them, had fewer worries, fewer personal problems and fewer practical needs on the second than on the first assessment.

The only statistically significant movement occurring within the comparison group was the reduction in practical needs between the first and second assessment.

Significant Differences in Movement Between the Two Groups. Practically all the signficant movements within the special group led to a significant difference in movement between the groups. There was one addition: significantly fewer clients deteriorated to the 'seriously ill' category in the special than in the comparison group.

In addition to these significant differences we noted many movements and differences in outcome, small in range, which consistently favoured the special group but which could nevertheless have occurred by chance. However, since with very few exceptions these differences went in the same direction it suggests a trend which could show up more definitely in a larger sample of old people.

In most respects we were able to see a correspondence between the input reported by the social workers and the outcome reported by the clients or judged by the independent assessors. However, when we consider the very considerable differences in the quantity and quality of social work performed by the workers in the two groups, it is perhaps a little disappointing that positive changes in outcome were few and mostly of small size.

Reference
Rieseman, David (1961): *The Lonely Crowd; a study of the Changing American Character*, Yale University Press.

7

INPUT AND OUTCOME IN RELATION TO INDIVIDUAL CASES

We now want to explore three sets of questions which concern the relationship between social work input and outcome in individual cases.

First: Did clients who had much help improve more than those who had little?

Second: Did clients who were judged by the assessors to have, initially, 'considerable' need for social work, improve more when helped by trained case workers than by social workers without professional training?

Third: Did clients with psychiatric conditions and with pronounced personal and interpersonal problems improve more under the care of trained social workers than with the help of those without professional training?

Individual Movement

In order to answer these questions one needed to assess the progress of *individual* cases between the first and the second assessment rather than to compare the two groups as a whole at two stages, which tells us little about the fate of individual clients.

It proved impossible to trace the progress of individual clients on all the 170 social and 143 medical assessments. It was necessary, therefore, to condense the material in such a way that those items which were highly related were grouped together. This statistical operation in which every item is correlated with every other was carried out using a computer (see Appendix 2), the final outcome being a 'component analysis'. This produced eleven 'factors' comprising items which hung together by virtue of their high intercorrelation (these factors are enumerated in Appendix 2). The results are interesting, as they show

how this mechanical operation will yield meaningful factors. For example, the items related to the mobility of the old people all came together in the same factor, whilst items concerned with, say, housing coalesced into another factor.

Having obtained these factors we then went back to the individual questionnaires to see how each client had scored on each factor. We calculated 'improvement' and 'deterioration' scores for each person on each factor. These scores were graded as follows:

'Significant'   improvement/deterioration=movement reaching significance level

'Considerable'   improvement/deterioration=less than significant but over 20 per cent change

'Some'   improvement/deterioration=10 per cent to 20 per cent change[1]

'No Change'   improvement/deterioration=less than 10 per cent change

The majority of people showed very little change on most factors; only two factors indicated significant change between first and second assessment, factors 4 and 3, the 'practical needs' factor and the 'morale' factor (see Appendix 2). This fits in with the findings reported in the last chapter where most of the differences between the groups clustered around two major areas – fulfilment of practical needs and subjective feelings of satisfaction, representing what may be called the 'morale' of the old people.

We therefore adopted the individual scores on the 'practical needs' and 'morale' factors as criteria of outcome to study the movement of individual clients during the course of the experiment.

Amount of Social Work and Outcome in Relation to Practical Needs
The 'practical needs' factor (factor 4) was derived from answers to questions about the total number of needs seen by the assessor, the number of social service needs, (this was a separate count) and the assessors' rating on 'indications for social work'. A significant number of clients in both groups improved markedly on their scores for the practical needs factor (Table VII. 1) but, as the table shows, individual

[1] No differences under 20 per cent were statistically significant.

TABLE VII. I

INDIVIDUAL CHANGES IN PRACTICAL NEEDS BASED ON FACTOR
SCORES

Amount of change in needs	Special group No. of clients	Comparison group No. of clients
Significant improvement	19	12
Considerable improvement	45	29
Some improvement	9	9
No change	31	40
Some deterioration	2	2
Considerable deterioration	3	9
Significant deterioration	1	3
	110	104

clients in the special group changed considerably more than clients in the comparison group. There were 23 more old people scoring considerable improvement or better in the special group, but eight fewer with 'considerable deterioration' or worse. When we related these positive and negative movements on the factor scores to the amount of social work done in each individual case, we saw a highly significant relationship (Table VII. 2).

For instance, among the 34 clients who had received 6 or more items of practical help 10 had a significantly improved score on reassessment (8 of these were in the special group) and no one in either group had deteriorated. At the other extreme, of the 94 who received very little practical help only 5 improved significantly (3 in the special and 2 in the comparison group) and 14 were worse off on second assessment (11 of these were in the comparison group). Relating individual changes in practical needs as measured by the factor scores to the number of visits paid we again see a close relationship (Table VII. 3).

Of the 83 clients who had 10 or more visits, only 2 had deteriorated at the second assessment (one in each group) and 20 had improved significantly. (15 of these were in the special group.) Of the 131 who had less than 10 visits, 18 were worse off on the second assessment (13 of these were in the comparison group) and only 11 had improved significantly (4 in the special and 7 in the comparison group).

Thus, the amount of social work done as measured by the number of contacts and amount of practical help is visibly related to a reduction in

TABLE VII. 2

INDIVIDUAL CHANGES IN NEEDS IN RELATION TO PRACTICAL HELP GIVEN

Number of items of practical help by social worker

Changes in needs	0–1			2–3			4–5			6+			Totals		
	SG*	CG*	Total	SG	CG	Total	SG	CG	Total	SG	CG	Total	SG	CG	Total
Significant improvement	3	2	5	5	5	10	3	3	6	8	2	10	19	12	31
Con./some improvement	17	19	36	6	12	18	13	7	20	18	0	18	54	38	92
No change	12	27	39	10	9	19	4	3	7	5	1	6	31	40	71
Deterioration	3	11	14	1	3	4	2	0	2	0	0	0	6	14	20
Totals	35	59	94	22	29	51	22	13	35	31	3	34	110	104	214

* SG = Special Group, CG = Comparison Group, notation used in subsequent tables.

TABLE VII. 3

INDIVIDUAL CHANGES IN NEEDS IN RELATION TO NUMBER OF VISITS

Number of visits

Changes in needs	0–4			5–9			10–14			15+			Totals		
	SG	CG	Total	SG	CG	Total	SG	CG	Total	SG	CG	Total	SG	CG	Total
Significant improvement	1	2	3	3	5	8	6	2	8	9	3	12	19	12	31
Con./some improvement	3	12	15	19	18	37	10	4	14	22	4	26	54	38	92
No change	3	14	17	12	21	33	8	2	10	8	3	11	31	40	71
Deterioration	0	6	6	5	7	12	1	0	1	0	1	1	6	14	20
Totals	7	34	41	39	51	90	25	8	33	39	11	50	110	104	214

practical needs as observed by an independent assessor who has no knowledge of what has actually been done by the social worker. It is worth noting that these relationships between input and outcome in individual cases are only statistically significant if we combine the special and comparison groups which then contain the whole range of social work input. They do not show up nearly as clearly within the separate groups because there was a general trend towards high input in the special group while the reverse was true in the comparison group.

Individual Changes in Morale and Amount of Social Work Done

The picture is not nearly as clear cut if we study the individual changes that occurred in the two groups in relation to the morale factor (Table VII. 4). This factor contained answers to questions about what the old people felt about life at the moment, whether anything worried them, whether they felt lonely and also judgements by the social work assessor on their contentment and personal problems (see Appendix 2).

TABLE VII. 4

INDIVIDUAL CHANGES IN MORALE BASED ON FACTOR SCORES

Amount of change in morale	Special group No. of clients	Comparison group No. of clients
Significant improvement	4	4
Considerable improvement	14	8
Some improvement	18	12
No change	65	67
Some deterioration	8	7
Considerable deterioration	0	5
Significant deterioration	1	1
	110	104

Although the differences in movement between the old people in the two groups were less marked the clients in the special group did better than the old people in the comparison group. Eighteen clients in the special group improved significantly and considerably in morale compared with 12 in the comparison group; and at the lower end of the distribution the differences were more pronounced. Six clients deteriorated significantly or considerably on the morale factor in the comparison group, compared with only 1 in the special group.

When we relate improvement in morale to the number of visits and items of practical help given to the individual clients, the relationships were not nearly as marked as those associated with the practical needs factor (Tables VII. 5 and VII. 6). Although there was a trend towards an association between the number of visits paid and improvement in morale it was not statistically significant. Improvement on the morale factor appeared to be more related to the amount of practical help given and to joining a club in the last ten months, particularly in the special group. For example, of the 30 clients who improved considerably or significantly in morale 12 had six or more items of practical help (all in the special group) and of the 22 who deteriorated only 2 had this amount of practical help.

Some Case Examples of Significant Improvement and Deterioration in 'Morale'
Other factors which we were unable to measure may influence morale, such as the quality of the client-worker relationship, the client's personality and other important changes in the clients' life situation, as we can see when we study some actual cases. For this we chose the case in each group which had scored highest on morale improvement and the case in each group which had deteriorated most from first to second assessment.

Improvement in Morale. We found that the case which had scored the greatest movement on the morale factor in the special group was that of Mrs A., a widow aged seventy-six referred to the welfare department by her daughter for no specified reason. She lived on social security and supplementary benefit in a damp basement flat of a condemned house without a bath or inside lavatory. A married daughter with her family and an unmarried son were occupying the upper part of the house. On first assessment Mrs A. was able to do most things for herself, although the medical assessor found her to be suffering from arteriosclerotic disease of the brain, manifesting as Parkinsonism, and from severe generalized osteo-arthritis. Mrs A. had a home help once a week but cooked her own meals; she did not belong to any clubs and said that sometimes 'I wander about from the garden to the front and I don't know what to do with myself'. She was dissatisfied with her life at the moment. The assessor summed up at the end of her interview: 'She is a very depressed old lady, she says she suffers from arthritis and evidently does

TABLE VII. 5

INDIVIDUAL CHANGES IN MORALE IN RELATION TO NUMBER OF VISITS

| Change in morale | Number of visits | | | | | | | | | | | | Totals | | |
| | 0–4 | | | 5–9 | | | 10–14 | | | 15+ | | | | | |
	SG	CG	Total	SG	CG	Total	SG	CG	Total	SG	CG	Total	SG	CG	Total
Sig./Con. improvement*	0	3	3	5	7	12	5	2	7	8	0	8	18	12	30
Some improvement*	2	5	7	8	5	13	3	1	4	5	1	6	18	12	30
No change	5	22	27	20	35	55	15	2	17	25	8	33	65	67	132
Deterioration	0	4	4	6	4	10	2	3	5	1	2	3	9	13	22
Totals	7	34	41	39	51	90	25	8	33	39	11	50	110	104	214

* As there were so few with significant improvements and a sizeable group with 'some' improvement, we have had to combine the 'significant' group with the 'considerable' group.

TABLE VII. 6

INDIVIDUAL CHANGES IN MORALE IN RELATION TO PRACTICAL HELP GIVEN

| Change in morale | Number of items of practical help by social worker | | | | | | | | | | | | Totals | | |
| | 0–1 | | | 2–3 | | | 4–5 | | | 6+ | | | | | |
	SG	CG	Total	SG	CG	Total	SG	CG	Total	SG	CG	Total	SG	CG	Total
Sig./Con. improvement*	2	7	9	4	3	7	0	2	2	12	0	12	18	12	30
Some improvement*	11	7	18	3	2	5	2	2	4	2	1	3	18	12	30
No change	19	41	60	12	16	28	18	9	27	16	1	17	65	67	132
Deterioration	3	4	7	3	8	11	2	0	2	1	1	2	9	13	22
Totals	35	59	94	22	29	51	22	13	35	31	3	34	110	104	214

See footnote, Table VII. 5.

not feel well, complaining of pains in her head, stomach upsets and trembling. She obviously feels very neglected by all her children. Her daughter is out at work all day and she says she only comes down a few times in the week to collect the shopping list and is in such a hurry that Mrs A. can never remember what she needs. The other children rarely come. She says she is very unhappy in the house and looks forward to it coming down and herself being rehoused. What she most dislikes is being on her own all day and rehousing would not solve this problem. She relates her state of depression to the fact that she is now housebound and unable to get out on her own. She gives the impression, however, that her unhappiness is of longer standing. The need is for a full assessment with reference to her doctor; can anything be done for the aches and pains she complains of?' The assessor considered that attendance at a day centre would be desirable and that social work contacts with relatives would be valuable. The assessor felt that Mrs A. could benefit greatly from more social contacts and some attention to her depressed state, but that this would depend partly on her physical health.

The social worker gave Mrs A., who was of very limited intelligence and very self-absorbed, without any kind of social stimulation, a great deal of practical help and support. She paid altogether 19 visits during the 10 months, contacted 10 different agencies on behalf of Mrs A. and also kept in touch with various members of Mrs A.'s family. In close collaboration with the general practitioner she arranged an examination by a geriatrician who recommended clearance of her teeth. Much encouragement was needed before Mrs A. was ready to have this done. The social worker accompanied her to the dental appointments and helped the dentist in coping with Mrs A.'s anxieties; she arranged for an eye examination, glasses and regular chiropody, from which she received great relief as her feet had not been attended to for 2 years. She introduced her to a club, to a voluntary visitor and arranged a holiday for her. The social worker's summary on handing the case back to the welfare department says: 'morale much better but need for further improvement in self-confidence and initiative. Mrs A. enjoys attendance at the centre and is on the waiting list for a second day per week. Introduced to a new club for physically handicapped and a voluntary visitor. Holiday, the first for many years, proved to be a great success – brought client much happiness and increased self-confidence. Casework aimed at enriching Mrs A.'s life by improved health and social contacts and by trying to improve her morale and self esteem; support given to family in their care of her, helping them to accept her limitations. Interpretation and liaison necessary with family, doctor, club; ventilation needed for client's and family's feelings. Mrs A. responds to support of caseworker, she has limited intelligence, is quickly deflated and needs much more support and appreciation from family and others. Should continue attendance at centre; support from regular contacts with social worker should aim at ensuring this, interpreting her needs and supplying aids and services as required.'

On her return visit after 10½ months the assessor who had no access to the first assessment report and was unaware of the social work carried out or the social worker's final summary, reports as follows at the end of her interview. 'Mrs A. was feeling extremely cheerful when I called, having three days previously returned from a holiday through the welfare department at Clacton. She spent a lot of time talking about her first experience of a holiday and had obviously thoroughly enjoyed herself. Her daily needs are covered by home help and a daughter living on first floor of house. Housing is poor and unsuitable. Mrs A. complains of loneliness as she is on her own all day but has now started attending a day centre and enjoys this. Mrs A. mentioned a lot of activities initiated by her social worker – dentist, glasses, holiday. In the client's own words "she's not bad, she does her best, fixed the holiday, took me to have teeth out, arranged to have eyes done".'

The medical assessor reported that her Parkinsonism had progressed rapidly between assessments; on the second occasion she was salivating, her tongue was rolling, her musculature rigid and her face mask-like. Her osteo-arthritis, especially of the hips and knees rendered her virtually immobile, though she was able to shuffle very slowly and painfully with the aid of a walking stick. She complained that 'everybody had let her down except Miss H.'

The case which scored most improvement on the morale factor in the comparison group was Mrs B., an eighty-year-old widow living alone in a ground-floor flat without an indoor lavatory or hot water. She was referred to the welfare department following discharge from a convalescent home by her general practitioner because she was housebound on account of her osteo-arthritis. She could wash and dress herself only with difficulty, and a home help had been provided five times a week by the time the assessor saw Mrs B. Her three sons visited weekly and she saw a great deal of her neighbour upstairs. The assessor comments:

'Her main problem to which she constantly referred is her loneliness. Her visit to the convalescent home, a positive experience, appears to have decided her she would like to go into a home. She did umbrella-making at home which she kept up to the age of seventy-nine. The end of this work and being housebound now seem to be the main factors in her loneliness. She was not willing to think of other ways of dealing with loneliness – clubs, etc., as her main desire is to "get out of it". She feels rehousing would be no solution since she would be as lonely. On the other hand she seems to envisage having a room to herself and possibly taking her own furniture to the home and I wondered if she had really given thought to what is involved. Social work help needed to discuss best solution with her. The absence of an ideal solution for Mrs B. e.g. a home to which she can take her own furniture, may make her difficult to help. She would, however, benefit in morale by having someone with whom she could explore all possibilities.'

The medical assessor reported that she was suffering from gross osteo-arthritis of knees and hips and congestive heart failure which was controlled by drugs. She also had had a mild stroke resulting in loss of power in her legs.

Mrs B. had the help of three different social workers from the welfare department who paid 8 visits in the 10 months and whose main aim was to help her to clarify and then to proceed with her plans to go into a residential home. Mrs B. talked freely about how she felt and was described as a sensible and friendly person who liked people. However, when eventually a vacancy was offered in a double room of a small home she could not face this and refused the offer. It then appeared that she was managing quite happily with the help of the home help, her neighbour upstairs and her neighbour next door who looked in every day. Also her health was better, she felt, and rails had been fixed (by a friend) all along the walls of her home. The social worker who had seen most of Mrs B. was also inclined to think that her health had improved and that Mrs B. was psychologically less dependent.

The second assessment took place shortly after Mrs B. made the decision, which she discussed at length with the social worker, not to go into a home. Asked how she had been getting on since last seen she said: 'Pretty fair, thank you. I can't get out but my health has been quite good'. The write-up at the end of the questionnaire is as follows: 'Mrs B. is a fairly contented person and says her health is good apart from the osteo-arthritis which keeps her housebound. She seems lonely

in spite of her home help every morning and a neighbour every afternoon and I felt she could be interested in going out to a day centre, but
she said she had never heard of these. She might also like a holiday or,
alternatively, the provision of transport facilities to friends in Clacton
where she went regularly on holiday when she could make the coach
journey. Asked me about almshouses where there is a matron who
goes round to see the old people are all right. She sub-lets the upstairs to
a widower who is very good to her, though at work all day, and her
married sons visit every week.'

Asked about social-work help she said she had various young ladies
who did not give her their names, but as she needed nothing they could
not help. She was very pleased about an unexpected Ministry of Social
Security grant of £5 for sweaters.

The medical assessor considered that her condition had altered little
between the assessment, 'She tended to play down the extent of her
disability'.

The greater contentment of Mrs A. and Mrs B. did not only come out
in the answers to the questions about satisfaction with life at the
moment, attitudes to the outside world, worries, loneliness and in the
assessor's judgement of personal problems but can also be understood
in terms of what had happened to Mrs A. and Mrs B. and of the general
impression conveyed during the second assessment interview. Mrs
A.'s improvement in morale is almost certainly related to the intensive
and continuous support and understanding this rather deprived and
simple woman received from her social worker and to the socially
enriching experiences the client enjoyed as a result of social work,
despite her apparent deterioration in her physical condition.

Mrs B.'s improvement in morale was possibly associated with her
better state of health and with working through the problem of whether
to go to a home, ending in a positive decision to make the best of her
life at home, while not losing the possibility of residential care later on.
It is of interest that none of the alternative avenues had been explored
for making Mrs B.'s life less monotonous and socially more stimulating.
(Some months later she asked for a holiday and for a day centre, while
still considering the possibility of going into a home.)

Deterioration in Morale. The only case in the special group which
scored significant deterioration on the morale factor was Mrs C., aged
seventy-three, living with her very ailing husband in a ground-floor flat

with no bathroom, hot water or indoor lavatory. She was very active, going out shopping every day and still taking on baby-minding. The couple was referred by their son when they both had bronchitis and needed a home help. The assessor described Mrs C. as an active, occupied, fairly happy person, possibly given to bouts of anxiety, who could probably manage as long as she was fit and active. The real problem was Mr C. (also in the study) who was registered as a physically handicapped person with chronic bronchitis and damage to his left leg as a result of an industrial accident. The medical assessor described Mrs. C. as a fit, active woman with a life-long history of neurotic traits.

This couple received and asked for a great deal of active casework, as massive problems, both practical and psychological were revealed. Mrs C., the dominant partner of a 'niggling and dependent' husband, was a heavy drinker; their marital conflict became more and more obvious; Mr C. deteriorated in health and was admitted to hospital with a multiplicity of complaints. Services such as meals-on-wheels and home help were provided from time to time and liaison with the hospital personnel maintained. Both husband and wife made much use of the caseworker in discussing their feelings and conflicts and depended on him a great deal. Support was also sought by their son who had his own marital problems.

The social worker felt that this was a challenging case and that the situation fluctuated according to the husband's condition. He thought that things might have got even worse without social work help.

When the social work assessor asked Mrs C. on her second visit how she had been getting on, she replied: 'Awful really. My husband's health worries me very much – the hospital keep saying he is coming home – I'm worried about it . . .', etc. The assessor comments at the end of the interview: 'Over and above the crisis of breakdown in Mr C.'s health, his doubtful future and the problems of his care, this situation is strongly coloured by a marital problem. Things seem bleak to Mrs C. She is controlling, and something like the possibility of Mr C. getting beyond her ministrations is very disturbing to her. She also longs to have another child to mind, yet feels doubtful whether she should. They need continued casework help particularly in resettling Mr C. at home. In view of his illness, her inability to cope and their relationship, the situation may not last long, even with massive support.' Mrs C. mentioned the regular visits of the social worker, 'I like to see him, someone to talk to; I want to see him now about Mr C. coming home.'

The medical assessor reported that Mrs C's health had not altered, but that her agitation had intensified because she was faced with the prospect of nursing her husband through a terminal illness. Her general practitioner was prescribing daily sedatives for her and sleeping tablets.

The client who deteriorated most on the morale factor in the comparison group was a widow, aged eighty-three, living alone in a rented ground-floor flat without a bath or inside lavatory. She was failing in sight and had been referred by her neighbour on account of her bad sight and loneliness. She was able to do most things for herself except heavy housework and washing and found difficulty in cooking herself a hot meal. Home help was provided twice a week and meals-on-wheels three times. She had no children, but received some visits from a niece and nephew and had contacts with helpful neighbours. She claimed never to be lonely and to be satisfied at the moment. 'At the age of eighty-three you don't expect anything different; a club would make a big difference, I like people.' The assessor comments 'She gives the impression of being a cherished neighbour and aunt; she has not got many problems – neighbours and friends help her. Needing help to get flat redecorated, and was enthusiastic about the possibility of a holiday. Appreciative of recent visits from welfare department and warmed to the possibility of a club. She should make good use of appropriate services and concern from a social worker. I imagine her old friends like her to be the gay and plucky old lady, but Mrs D. indicated anxiety about eyesight, health and being alone.'

The medical assessor describes Mrs D. as 'a small, frail but mobile woman, slightly forgetful and repetitious, low in morale and expressing, on both occasions a wish to be dead. Her vision was impaired by cataracts and macula degeneration. She was chronically constipated and slept only with the aid of barbiturates. She smoked 15 cigarettes a day.'

One social worker from the welfare department supported this old lady throughout; she was in touch with many organizations on her behalf, including her general practitioner, the club organizer and the old peoples' welfare committee. She arranged aids, chiropody and a club for her and felt that the old lady appreciated any help and support she could give her. At the end of the experimental period the social worker considered that there was slight improvement due to the supporting services and the social contacts at the club. However she also felt that the client was going downhill physically and becoming increasingly unable to cope.

When on the second assessment visit the social work assessor inquired how she had been getting on in the intervening period, Mrs D. said: 'Oh, all right. I've got some wonderful friends. But when you get my age, you don't want to bother with anything – I get so depressed.' The assessor wrote at the end of her interview: 'Mrs D. has deteriorated considerably since I last saw her, mainly in a physical sense; she looks grubby and not very well kempt, is a bit incontinent of faeces at night; she also seems to be finding everything a bit beyond her; is spending a good deal of time in bed and is no longer buying food on the scale that she was. She appears to be thinner.' The assessor felt that Mrs D. would welcome a discussion about an old peoples' home, as things were getting too much for her. She was inclined to wish she were dead because of her loneliness and her increasing infirmity; she was glowing in her praise of welfare services though she did not seem to link them in any way with her social worker. In answer to the question whether she had found the visits a help she was not sure but said, 'there is nothing she can do, I am sure she would if she could'. In answer to what she felt about life at the moment she said 'I've got to put up with it, I wish I were dead. I pray for it every night, I want to be with my husband but I have got to put up with it.' This lady's wish was soon fulfilled; she died two months later.

It seems that in both cases in which significant deterioration in morale had taken place, circumstances beyond the social workers' control had worsened: in one instance a serious crisis was overwhelming an already chronically disturbed alcoholic woman, in the other case physical deterioration seems to have led to an acceleration of 'disengagement' and profound depression in someone who perhaps had shown too 'plucky' a face to the outside world previously.

The four examples show how complex the relationships are between expressed attitudes, summed up in the concept of an old person's morale, her personality and her life situation which includes her health and the help and support she is receiving. What seems to stand out most in this descriptive analysis of the best and worst cases in relation to improvement in morale is how strongly physical well-being impinges on morale in old age. All three of those over seventy-five (Mrs A., B., & D.) were preoccupied with their health and aware of their helplessness in face of growing disability and incapacity. Yet all three were still able to respond to socially stimulating and supportive influences coming from outside. Mrs A., though hardly able to move with osteo-arthritis and handicapped by severe Parkinsonism, had the time of her life on her first holiday at the age of seventy-six. Even Mrs D. still cherished her club to which the social worker had introduced her and left her bed to go there once a week.

Relationship between Need for Social Work and Outcome

We now want to consider the second question concerned with the relationship between input and outcome in individual cases.

Did the clients who were judged by the assessors to have, initially, 'considerable' need for social work, improve more when helped by trained case workers than by social workers without professional training?

It has been shown in Chapter VI that those in the special group considered to be most in need of social work by the assessors had twice as much help on average as those whose needs were considered slight. In the comparison group this trend was not so marked. It could be argued that trained social workers will be able to use their skills to the fullest degree with clients whose need for social work was considerable and who had many and complex problems. Among this group were old people with severe personal or psychiatric problems, such as depression and confusion, those with severe physical disabilities combined with housing problems and interpersonal stresses and those with difficult family situations.

In order to test the proposition that the trained caseworkers would achieve better results with this difficult group of clients, we related the indications for social work as judged by the assessors at the beginning of the case to the outcome, as measured by improvement on the need and morale factors. The results are presented in Tables VII.7 and VII.8. They are of great interest, as the picture is very different for changes in practical needs and for improvement in morale. Looking at the clients whose need for social work was considerable we find that roughly the same proportions in the special and comparison group, namely just over two-thirds, were found to have reduced practical needs at the end of the experiment (Table VII. 7). This was achieved although the social workers in the comparison group visited less often than the project social workers and gave less practical help. However, scrutiny of the comparison group cases which improved revealed that they were visited on average fourteen times during this ten-month period, which

TABLE VII. 7

INDIVIDUAL CHANGES IN 'NEEDS' IN RELATION TO INDICATIONS FOR SOCIAL WORK

Indications for social work	Changes in needs in special group				Changes in needs in comparison group			
	Improved §	*No change*	*Deteriorated*	*Total*	*Improved* §	*No change*	*Deteriorated*	*Total*
Slight	20	21	2	43	11	28	4	43
Moderate	29	15	1	45	21	20	7	48
Considerable	15	5	1	21	9	3	1	13
Totals	64	41	4	109*	41	51	12	104

* One old person in the special group was not rated on indications for social work.
§ 'Improved' here relates to significant and considerable improvement.

TABLE VIII. 8

INDIVIDUAL CHANGES IN 'MORALE' IN RELATION TO INDICATIONS FOR SOCIAL WORK

Indications for social work	Changes in 'morale' in special group				Changes in 'morale' in comparison group			
	Improved §	*No change*	*Deteriorated*	*Total*	*Improved* §	*No change*	*Deteriorated*	*Total*
Slight	1	41	1	43	1	42	0	43
Moderate	8	37	0	45	10	33	5	48
Considerable	9	12	0	21	1	11	1	13
Totals	18	90	1	109*	12	86	6	104

* One old person in the special group was not rated on indications for social work.
§ 'Improved' here relates to significant and considerable improvement.

is a much higher average than for cases in the comparison group as a whole.

Looking at the clients with 'considerable' need for social work in relation to improvement in morale, we find a very different picture. Nearly half the special group cases improved 'considerably' and 'significantly' (9 out of 21) but only 1 out of 13 in the comparison group. Where the indications for social work were 'moderate' or 'slight' we could detect no difference in outcome between the two groups. We realize that numbers are very small and dictate great caution in the interpretation of these results. Nevertheless the suggestion emerges that the social workers in the comparison group were just as capable of solving the practical problems of their most complex cases as were the trained workers, but they were less able to bring about improvement in the more intangible dimensions of feelings and attitudes.

Outcome in Relation to Psychiatric and Personal Problems
The medical assessor originally considered that 46 clients had a serious psychiatric disorder (Chapter III, p. 169). Of these 30 were suffering from severe organic brain syndrome (15 in each group). Only just over half (16 out of the 30) were still living in their own home at the end of the experiment – 6 in the special and 10 in the comparison group; 8 had died (4 in each group), a much higher proportion than in the group as a whole (27 per cent compared with 16 per cent). Five of the special group clients suffering from organic brain syndrome had gone into hospital or into a residential home, but only one in the comparison group. There is a suggestion here, confirmed by a study of these cases, that the social workers in the special group were more active in obtaining residential care for their most confused clients who could no longer hold their own in the community.

The situation is quite different for the 16 clients who were initially diagnosed as suffering from functional disorder. Twelve of the 16 were still at home on reassessment (9 out of 11 in the special group and 3 out of 5 in the comparison group), 3 had died and 1 had gone into hospital. These proportions are almost identical with the proportions dying, going into institutions and staying at home in the sample as a whole. As was noted in Chapter III (p. 72) most of these functional disturbances had become stabilized and the old people and perhaps their relatives and friends too, had learned to live with them. Although the project social workers recognized most of the functional psychiatric problems diagnosed by the medical assessor and were in close touch with the general practitioner about some of them, only one was seen by a psychiatrist.

When we examined the individual improvement of all clients who had been diagnosed as having any psychiatric trouble (38 in the special and 28 in the comparison group) we found that more had improved, both, in morale and in relation to their practical needs in the special group, than in the comparison group, but the numbers involved are too small to draw any general conclusion. It is worth noting that (in both groups) the amount of improvement among the psychiatrically disturbed clients was similar to that prevailing in the groups as a whole and that the number of visits paid and the amount of practical help given was also very near to the general average. Thus psychiatric disturbance *per se* did not seem to be a crucial consideration in relation to social work effort or outcome. Of greater relevance seemed to be whether these psychiatric disturbances express themselves in personal problems and in interaction with others. For if we look at those old people who in the opinion of the assessors had pronounced personal and interpersonal problems, then we find that the social workers in the special group were able to bring about considerably more improvement both on the practical and especially on the morale level, than did the social workers of the other group. Most of these clients with severe personal and interpersonal problems were judged to be in considerable need of social work and we have already seen that the project social workers achieved more improvement in morale in this particularly demanding group of cases.

In summary, we have shown that the input of social work is related to outcome in individual cases, particularly in the more measurable practical sphere. In the more intangible fields of feelings and attitudes we have not been able yet to identify clearly the input ingredients responsible for any results achieved. Individual case examples showed the complex interaction between expressed feelings and attitudes, summed up in the concept of morale, and the clients' personality and life situation in which physical well-being plays a large part and which includes the help and support received from social workers.

Looking more closely at those clients whose problems were manifold and complex a suggestion emerged that while the social workers with good experience and considerable specialist knowledge can achieve as much as their fully trained social work colleagues in meeting practical needs, professionally trained social workers appear to achieve more in meeting subjective and psychological needs than those who have not had training in differential casework methods.

8

THE CONSUMERS' OPINION

So far we have compared the clients' answers to questions about their social and medical conditions, their physical and social functioning, their attitudes and feelings, at the beginning and at the end of the experiment. We detected some changes in their answers, particularly among the clients in the special group and concluded that these changes were related to the social work effort. What were the clients' own views on the services they were offered? In this chapter we want to explore what the clients themselves thought about the help they had received. At the end of the reassessment interview the old people answered several questions about their contacts with social workers and their comments were recorded verbatim. The social assessors also noted clients' comments and attitudes about the social work and the welfare services in their narrative.

The clients' reactions to the opening questions the assessors asked on their second visit are also relevant to the consumer aspects of this study. To the first question 'Do you remember me?' about three-quarters of the clients in both groups replied in the affirmative and the rest were either 'not sure' or said that they did not recall the visit. The differences between the groups were slight and in striking contrast to their recall and perceptions of the social workers which revealed highly significant differences between the groups, as we shall show below. To the second inquiry 'How have you been getting on since I saw you last?' around 73 per cent of the clients in both groups replied that they felt the same and only 14 per cent in each group said that they felt better, while about 10 per cent thought that they felt worse. On first sight these responses are somewhat disappointing when one considers the magnitude and intensity of the social work effort. The verbatim comments of the old people make it clear that the majority interpreted this question in terms of physical well-being, mobility and capacity to do everyday things and only a very small proportion, around 10 per cent, mentioned other important events in their lives, such as bereavements. Another rather general question, whether they had anybody with whom they could talk things over also failed to register any impact from their contacts with social workers; the clients usually mentioned relatives and friends and only one or two referred to a social worker.

Recall of Visits

Interesting and important differences between the two groups began to emerge when the clients were asked more specifically about the social workers' visits, how regular they had been and how much help they had derived from them. To the first question, whether a welfare officer had called during the past year, 95 per cent in the special group replied in the affirmative but only 77 per cent in the comparison group. Since everybody had been visited at least once or twice we examined more closely the situations of the five clients in the special group and the 20 clients in the comparison group who denied having had a visitor at all.

In the special group we did not have far to look for explanations. All five clients had been 'failures' both from the client's and the social worker's point of view. In their final evaluation questionnaire the social workers had marked all these cases as 'difficult to help'. Among them was an old lady who had been visited 21 times, but who was grossly deluded and confused and could not be persuaded by psychiatrist, general practitioner or social worker to take her tablets or to contemplate any other form of treatment. The second of the five was the eccentric recluse (discussed in some detail in Chapter V, p. 117) who insisted on shutting out the social worker and any other social contacts. In the remaining three cases clients expressed negative opinions about the social workers, partly because the help they had sought was not forthcoming. One old woman whose house was condemned and scheduled to come down in the near future was completely preoccupied with her rehousing problem. The social worker's efforts with the housing authorities were of no avail and the client refused to contemplate any temporary improvements in her home. In another case of tragi-comedy endless troubles developed over supplying a wheelchair which engendered many difficulties and bitter feelings on the part of the client. In the fifth instance the social worker attempted to brighten the lives of a rather odd isolated couple – a suspicious spinster who was living with an elderly mentally-handicapped god-daughter – with somewhat disastrous results. They very much wanted a television set. The social worker, exercising considerable ingenuity, was able to produce one. But the two ladies became convinced that electricity was emanating from the set and it had to be removed. The clients lost confidence in the social worker, indeed they mistrusted him and he felt unable to repair the damage caused to the relationship.

In short, all these five clients appeared unable to recall what had been a frustrating experience for them. It is very unlikely that they did not remember the social workers who had taken great pains to reach them and meet their expressed needs. The social workers on their part felt defeated and rebuffed at the end of their endeavours and found it difficult to persevere in the face of their clients' lack of response or rejection of them; yet these people may have been the very ones who needed help most.

The situation is less clear among the 20 clients in the comparison group who said that they had had no visits. Six of them were only visited once or twice, but 14 had between 3 and 7 visits. As in the special group, for some of these 14 clients the experience of social work seems to have been a somewhat negative one, the client feeling that his needs, as he saw them, had not been recognized. An aggravating factor in the situation may have been that only 3 of these 14 old people had the same worker throughout. In some cases, where several social workers moved in and out of the clients' lives, they had not really established any contact with the old person. For example a few old people who had experienced bereavement needed more intensive and continuous support from one sympathetic person. One old man said sadly to the assessor: 'In view of my dear wife's death I just live from day to day. I am completely absorbed with the thoughts of my wife not being with me.' Other clients, though under considerable stress did not voice any specific complaints or requests for services. They needed skilful help in exploring their problems. For instance one housebound lady of eighty-six whose health was deteriorating after a stroke was being looked after by her niece aged seventy-three. This niece, although uncomplaining, was feeling the strain and needed practical help and encouragement. Another client who felt unhelped said: 'I have not got the "push" for clubs'. She felt unwell with 'nerves' and was worried about her neighbour moving away, adding: 'I've got to be satisfied with life.' A feeling of resignation, of being forgotten and not cared for runs through many of the comments. A few clients seemed to connect the visits with the possibility of 'being put in a home' and were fearful about this. Changes of social worker made it perhaps more difficult to confide their fears, although they did feel able to mention them to the assessors.

In contrast to the project social workers who had recorded that all five clients who denied being visited had been difficult to help, the social workers in the comparison group only found 4 of the 20 difficult to help. While the social workers in the special group thought that 1 of the 5 had improved and 3 were worse off at the end of their endeavours, the social workers in the comparison group considered that 13 of the 20 had improved and none were worse at the end of the experiment. It seems that the social workers without professional training did not always recognize the complexities and difficulties presented by clients who 'forgot' that they had ever been visited by a social worker.

Regularity of Visiting

Eighty per cent of the clients in the special group said that they had had regular visits compared with 41 per cent in the comparison group. According to the information supplied by the social workers 93 per cent of the clients in the special group and 67 per cent in the comparison group had been visited at least 5 times, that is to say once in two months. It will be noted that the old people's estimate comes much closer to the recorded entries of the social workers' in the special than in the comparison group. This may again be related to the continuity of contact in the special group and possibly also to the project workers' greater perception of need and their skill in forging a fruitful relationship. The clients' recall of visits which took place at least once a month was also much more accurate in the special than in the comparison group. Sixty-six old people in the special group and 21 clients in the comparison group said that they had been visited once a month or oftener. Comparing these statements with the social workers' records we find complete agreement in 44 of these cases in the special group but in only 8 cases in the comparison group (Table VIII. 1).

How Help was Perceived

The question whether the old people had found the visits a help yielded interesting and revealing comments. Seventy-seven per cent of those who acknowledged having visits in the special group had found them

TABLE VIII. I

WELFARE CLIENTS' AND SOCIAL WORKERS' REPORTS ON
MONTHLY VISITING

Number of welfare clients reporting visits at least once a month	Special group 66	Comparison group 21
Of These social worker reports visits		
Once a month or oftener (10 +)	44	8
Approximately once a month (8 or 9)	13	5
Less than once a month (7 or less)	9	8

'helpful' compared with 48 per cent in the comparison group, statistically a highly significant difference.

Asked for their reasons, around half (52 per cent in the special and 45 per cent in the comparison group) made positive comments about the social workers and their relationships with them. These comments were almost always interspersed with appreciative references to practical help received.

In the special group, where contact was more regular and with one worker only, the comments were longer and conveyed more warmth and colour, reflecting, at times in humorous ways, the personalities of the two case workers: 'If I want anything, she'll get it; she is a dear, as good as your own; the welfare are very good.'

'Shan't half be sorry when he goes to Oxford – he said he'll come and see me; I like him very much; do anything for me. M. is a champion, would have done a lot more if I had let him, a very willing sort of chap. Made appointments for me with my G.P. Been on to me about a holiday.'

'She's a woman who gets things done – she's got a mind! She's got me a gas fire and she wants me to go to the centre. She got me an armchair. She's a very capable woman. She's had an awful job to get the gas. Very nice woman.' (At the medical reassessment this man called the doctor's attention to the very efficient gas fire obtained for him.)

'I notice the difference with all the help I'm getting now. Sometimes twice a month – he never misses. Have a long chat – have some rare talks with him. He got me the home help and wrote to my regiment for television and transistor. They couldn't do any more for me.'

'Arranged centre and a holiday. She's sensible, you can say things to her you might not to some people.'

'He has a chat, takes me to the chiropodist and to the doctor, very good like that; he gave me his telephone number in case I needed him. That's why I am so contented, because I know someone will be here [home help] and I've got somebody coming.'

'If I wanted any help I should contact Miss H. and ask her who to apply to. Yes – we feel as though we are being looked after.'

'Oh yes – we have a chat – usually something to talk about to do with my welfare. He keeps an eye on me. Heaps of help, yes. If I didn't have a bad leg I wouldn't need any help. Sometimes I feel I'm too dependent on other people for my errands.'

'I like her calling, a bit of company, a dear. Occasionally, if anything occurred I'd ring her, such a nice person. Did all she could – a back rest for my husband and a bath seat; kept coming after my husband died. Took me to the chiropodist in her car; arranged meals on wheels.'

'I like him very much indeed. We have a good laugh and joke together. Said he'd do anything for me; wish he were not leaving. He's fixing a holiday. Looks like one of the Rolling Stones – very nice.' (At the medical reassessment this woman said to the doctor 'Mr P. is going. Oh! it's a pity. He's been so good – my *only* bit of recreation on a Thursday. It's an *awful* shame.')

'We didn't ask for nothing, it was her got the meter shifted and the coin meter put in.'

'Has not been for three weeks; sometimes came nearly every day; oh yes, he is an old woman, treated me like a father. Used to ask me if I wanted anything. Welfare people are wonderful, if I needed anything I've only got to get in touch with them.'

'Very nice indeed she is, got me a rubber mat and rubber sheet, helps me out of trouble. Got no complaints, gives me all I want.'

The appreciative comments in the comparison group were briefer, somewhat less personal and expressive and often referred to the social worker not 'coming back'.

'Ever such a nice lady, got a walking stick for my husband. Like a university lady she was.'

'She's very nice. She doesn't do anything to help but comes to see me.'

'Got me a pension and Christmas parcel.'

'Has a chat, offered help with holiday.'

'Very helpful, arranged the club and holiday, and help with move and transfer. Very nice person. Had she been here I would have asked her about redecorating, but she's gone off to the wilds, seen nobody since. Perhaps they think I am an independent type. But I am willing to accept help. She rang up about rehousing and said: "Don't accept anything you don't want".'

'Saw the doctor about a flat for me but she hasn't been back.'

'I can't do handicrafts, but I enjoy her coming.'

'I think she's being trained – only a young woman; she comes to see if I'm all right.'

'Very considerate woman, very good at Christmas.'

'Glad they keep an eye on me. I never mind visitors.'

'I forget so quickly. They came about a centre but no one has been since.'

'Got me a carrying chair. They would have got me a wheelchair if they possibly could. I've had several different ones and they have all been very nice.' (At the medical reassessment this client asked the doctor whether he could do anything to get her a walking frame.)

As the quotations show, most clients mentioned spontaneously some material help the social worker had arranged or tried to obtain for them. But many also stressed the value of 'just having a chat' and that it was reassuring to know that somebody was there if you needed them.

Not unexpectedly twice as many clients in the special group (53) mentioned practical help as in the comparison group (26) (Table VIII. 2). Holidays and clubs were mentioned most often in both groups.

TABLE VIII. 2

ITEMS OF PRACTICAL HELP SPONTANEOUSLY MENTIONED BY WELFARE CLIENTS

Type of help	Special group (N=53)	Comparison group (N=26)
Holidays and clubs	30	14
Services (social and medical)	21	6
Aids and appliances	21	6
Material goods	5	2
Personal escort	4	1
Financial help	4	3
Housing	4	3
	89*	35*

* Many clients in both groups mentioned more than one item of practical help.

It is remarkable that the clients in the special group referred to aids and appliances such as wheelchairs, bath seats, special gadgets, more than three times as often as the clients in the comparison group. It seems that these aids made much difference to the old people's lives, but unfortunately the assessors were not able to observe the existence of additional aids on their visits and we omitted to include a specific question about this aspect of practical help. In general the clients' spontaneous comments about the practical services which they had valued reflect the social workers' own emphases in their activities. (See especially Table V. 8 p. 115).

What permeates these positive comments above all is the pleasure about needs being met, both material and psychological, the feeling of being cared for and the sense of security arising from knowledge of where to turn in time of need.

Seven clients in the special group and twelve clients in the comparison group were candid and bold enough to say that the visits had been of no help to them. They constituted 7 per cent and 15 per cent respectively of those who acknowledged that they had been visited. A larger proportion – 16 per cent in the special and 35 per cent in the comparison group – preferred to be non-committal, saying that they were not sure whether the visits had been of any help to them. It seemed important to explore the possible reasons for the frankly negative reactions to the social workers' efforts.

They fall mainly into three groups.

First there were three clients, two in the comparison and one in the special group, who really did not need any help. For example a cheerful old lady in the comparison group who was surrounded by her family who cared for her with devotion said: 'They could see I was all right and looked after by my family.'

There were also the more acid comments of an old man in the special group who was devoted to his home help and who said that he was always glad to be visited by nice young ladies but 'I can see no point in people coming and asking a lot of questions and then leaving saying "Look after yourself", and coming in a car to tell you this.'

Secondly, there were the clients (six in the comparison and four in the special group) for whom the help they had been offered was not relevant to what they conceived to be their needs. For instance, an old lady in the comparison group who had been rehoused to a rather sumptuous flat from slum property would have liked a few additional pieces of furniture; and an old couple, also in the comparison group, lived in terror of a mentally-ill tenant who kept disturbing them – knocking at their door, and shouting sometimes in the middle of the night. They felt strongly that this tenant should have been removed. There was the frail old lady in the comparison group who relied heavily on a friend down the road. She had refused an offer of residential accommodation but clearly felt she would have liked to talk to someone about this. 'She would have got me in a home but I refused, and she hasn't been lately, she's gone away.' Another example of feeling unhelped was that of a rather embittered old lady in the comparison group who lived with her blind son. She said; 'It is just as well to be truthful, she was no help. They gave me two fireguards.' The assessor thought that her problems centred around her anxieties about her growing infirmities and her son's future and that this woman who felt neglected by the welfare services probably needed a social worker in her own right rather than as 'Bill's mother'. Another instance was someone in the special group who had to wait for transport to a club for almost 10 months. Yet another client in the special group, the father of a longstanding 'problem' family with chronic debts and complex family relationships said: 'I've not got much help from the welfare, they only ask how we're getting on and I want the gas put on; it would be better if one person always came. We've had no help except getting me to the clubs.' (This family had been visited regularly by one of the project social workers who gave them much practical and psychological support; clearly this man did not feel it made any difference.) An old man in the special group was very critical of the services for the elderly, mainly because he had been offered a holiday in May when as a bronchitic he considered he needed to go away in the summer. He also was annoyed that no one could tell him where to apply for a local charity pension. (Actually the social worker collected all the available information for him, but did not have it at his fingertips!) He felt that information of this kind should be widely publicized and that all welfare officers should know about it. He also thought that there should be some more systematic seeking out of elderly persons in need, for instance, he pointed out that had he not applied for meals-on-wheels and thereby come to the attention of the welfare department no one would have known of his existence. Another client in the special group replied to the question whether the visits had been of help: 'Oh she comes, has a little chat to see how you get on; she said she could send a school girl but I've got nothing to say to a school girl.' This woman also felt that the clubs were 'cliquish' and that one is ignored if one does not belong to a clique.

Lastly, there was a third group of rather difficult and at times seriously disordered personalities who refused help and who were difficult to reach. Two ladies in the comparison group were rather vague and confused and both of them eventually went into mental hospitals. Two other clients in the comparison group were somewhat isolated and independent; one of them, a widower had lost his wife in the preceding year and both these clients probably needed skilled casework to lower their defences and enable them to discuss their loneliness. Another example in the special group was an old lady of eighty who said sharply 'I've told him not to call.' The assessor wrote 'She is something of a witch who sits in the middle of an untidy room (which is crammed with furniture). She is large, very guarded about anything to do with her feelings or her contacts with people and very irritated by the questionnaire. At one point when I was probing about her family she burst into tears in spite of herself and said how fond she was of her sister and her grandchild. All this behind a firm denial that she is lonely. She refuses to admit to being in need of anything (e.g. home help, club, money, etc.) and says she does not want anyone to see her. She used to have a man call from the Town Hall but she asked him not to come any more as he was no help or use to her. Life and relationships are felt by Mrs Z. to have been unsatisfactory and she wants to rely on herself. She probably can't stand a conversation but might respond to practical and concrete help.'

This lady was, in fact, more unbalanced than became apparent to the assessor. She was at times very confused and paranoid and not long after the reassessment visit was admitted to hospital in a confused state.

Surveying the negative reactions to social work help we need not feel concern about the first group of clients who did not really require any help. It is possible that the third group of very disordered old people were not able to take advantage of social work help. This does not absolve social workers from ensuring that the clients are not discarded because they are 'difficult'. However, much can be learnt from the criticisms voiced in the second group, where the social workers failed to meet the needs as they were perceived by the clients. Some of these needs were apparently simple like the bits of furniture required when an aged person moves from a slum to a well appointed flat. Other needs were more concealed and required skill to recognize and deal with. Yet other problems such as the disturbance caused by the mentally-ill neighbour could not be resolved, however hard both the neighbour's mental welfare officer and the old couple's social worker tried. The situation raised more fundamental problems of the containment of the mentally ill in the community and the burden this may place on citizens.

It is instructive that yet another consumer question 'Do you feel you have had enough help in the past year' differentiated much less between the two groups and brought forth more stereotyped answers than the specific question about the helpfulness of the visits. Eighty per cent of the clients in the special and 68 per cent in the comparison group thought that they had had enough help, a considerably higher proportion than those who had found the visits helpful. It is possible that these conforming clients whose expectations were low responded to such general questions in a polite stereotype 'Thank you, I had enough help'. They may also have been dimly aware of their increasing dependence on the goodwill of the social services generally in their advancing years.

Additional Help
Finally we also asked the clients whether they thought that anything else could or should be done to help them.

To our surprise more people in the special than in the comparison group said 'yes' to this question (Table VIII. 3), despite their greater feelings of satisfaction which were evident, both in their answers to questions about worries, depression, satisfaction with life at the moment and in their comments on the helpfulness of the social workers. Could it be that their greater experience of concrete help and of a caring relationship and their resulting higher morale and confidence in themselves contributed to a rise in expectations and to a decrease in feelings of resignation which prompted them to 'put up with things'? If this is so then paradoxically more expressed need may be an encouraging result of this experiment.

In Summary
These old welfare clients were well aware of the meaning of regular support and consistent interest. They clearly expressed their pleasure and appreciation of both material and psychological support when it had met their felt needs. This happened significantly more often in the special group. When social work had failed to meet their needs they

TABLE VIII. 3

ADDITIONAL HELP DESIRED BY WELFARE CLIENTS

Type of Help	Special group (N=35)	Comparison group (N=27)
Aids	1	3
Chiropody	–	3
Christmas parcel	1	3
Clothing	1	3
Club	1	–
Dentures	–	1
Domiciliary services	5	3
Holiday	1	2
' Hospital/residential care	2	–
Money	8	1
Outings	2	1
Redecorating	3	2
Rehousing	8	9
TV	2	–
Visit from general practitioner	–	2
	35	33*

* Six clients in the comparison group mentioned two items of additional help.

either denied that they had ever been in contact with social workers or they expressed doubts and criticisms about their experiences with them.

Thus, even very old people whose expectations are low and whose memories are often impaired can tell us what it is they want and what makes them feel helped if we care to ask them.

PART IV

Summary and Conclusions

9

HELPING THE AGED

Conclusions and Reflections

Summary

In the preceding pages we described the results of a field experiment in social work among 300 old people aged seventy and over who were clients of a London Borough welfare department.

Their social and medical condition and needs were assessed by a social worker and a physician. Nearly half the applicants were over eighty and most had been resident in the area for more than 20 years; nearly half were living in unsuitable or inconvenient housing and two-thirds lived alone. Children and neighbours were in frequent contact with the old people and very few were socially isolated.

These welfare clients were more incapacitated than random samples studied in similar age groups in Britain. A quarter were suffering from a serious disease which constituted a threat to life and 15 per cent suffered from psychiatric disorders.

Considering their incapacity and age many of these clients were still relatively active. Nearly two-thirds got out at least once a week and a quarter belonged to clubs.

Half the sample were already receiving some personal social services before their contact with the welfare department which brought them into this experiment. The medical and social assessors uncovered many additional medical and social needs. Only 5 per cent appeared to be in need of residential care. These 300 welfare clients were randomly allocated to a special group and a comparison group, which proved to be reasonably well matched in all important respects, except that there were more men in the special group. Two trained caseworkers were appointed to take on the social work in the special group while the comparison group remained under the care of the department's welfare officers, none of whom had a professional social-work training. The amount and quality of the social work differed greatly in the two groups. The old people in the special group had twice the amount of help received by those in the comparison group where the social workers carried bigger caseloads. The trained workers saw more problems and laid more emphasis on casework and work with relatives. They worked more closely with medical and with voluntary agencies, and with volunteers; they made greater efforts to enrich their clients' lives by introducing them to clubs, encouraging holidays and outings and by drawing in volunteers. They worked more selectively according to people's needs.

After $10\frac{1}{2}$ months the social and medical assessors reassessed all the survivors remaining in their own homes – 110 in the special and 104 in the comparison group – on the same criteria as on the first occasion, not knowing who was in the special and comparison groups and not having access to their previous assessments. Few, if any changes had occurred in the clients' material living conditions. Not surprisingly with people of this age, the general health of both groups had deteriorated. Their mobility, their capacity to perform basic tasks of everyday living and contacts with relatives and neighbours had remained virtually the same. Both groups had significantly fewer practical needs on reassessment, but this was even more apparent among the clients in the special group. The clients in the special group had also improved significantly in their 'morale', more of them were attending clubs, had had a holiday, felt satisfied with life, had a positive attitude to the world around them, had fewer worries and personal problems. They were significantly more active and less depressed than the old people in the comparison group. In addition to these statistically significant differences we observed movements and differences in outcome, small in range, which consistently favoured the special group. In most respects we could see a close correspondence between the input reported by the social workers and the outcome reported by the clients or judged by the independent assessors.

Looking at outcome in individual cases it became evident that reduction in practical needs was significantly related to input as measured in number of contacts and items of practical help given. We were not able to identify with any precision the elements in the casework process which were responsible for changes in attitudes and feelings, although case examples of improvement and deterioration in clients' 'morale' threw some light on the complex interaction between their feelings and attitudes summed up in the concept of morale, their life situation, and the help and support received by social workers.

Testing the Hypotheses

How do these findings relate to the hypotheses formulated at the beginning of the study? We found that one of the three general hypotheses was partially upheld and five of the seven specific hypotheses were confirmed.

General Hypotheses

1. *'More clients in the special group will survive to the time of the second assessment than in the comparison group.'*

While fewer clients died in the special group this outcome was not statistically significant, but significantly fewer clients in the special group than in the comparison group deteriorated to the seriously ill category on *one* overall medical rating scale. These two findings together suggest a trend in the direction of the hypothesis.

2. *'More clients in the special group will show positive changes in their social and medical condition than in the comparison group.'*

This hypothesis was partially upheld.

We have shown that significantly more clients in the special group improved in various aspects of their social functioning and in relation to their practical needs. But the hypothesis was not upheld in regard to the medical condition of the old people, since on most of the varying medical measures both groups deteriorated about equally in their general health and also in relation to minor disabilities and discomforts.

3. *'Fewer clients in the special group will be admitted to institutional care than in the comparison group.'*

This hypothesis was not upheld since roughly equal proportions were in hospital and residential homes at the end of the experiment.

Specific Hypotheses

1. *'Fewer clients in the special group will show deterioration in scores for self-care and household capacity than in the comparison group.'*

This hypothesis was not upheld since neither group deteriorated markedly in scores for self-care and household capacity.

2. *'There will be no difference between the special and comparison group in relation to improved amenities, e.g., means of heating, toilet arrangements, cooking facilities, adaptations and aids.'*

This hypothesis was upheld in general since there was little difference between the groups in these respects. (The hypothesis could not be tested adequately as regards aids and adaptations; the indications are from the social workers' reports and the clients' spontaneous comments that many more aids and adaptations were supplied in the special group, thus disproving the hypothesis.)

3. *'More clients in the special than in the comparison group will have improved their social contacts with family, neighbours and friends.'*

This hypothesis was not upheld since neither group showed any significant improvement in their contacts with family, neighbours and friends.

4. *'More people in the special than in the comparison group will develop interests and activities, e.g. clubs, work groups, holidays, home library, church contacts, hobbies.'*

This hypothesis was upheld in several respects; significantly more old people in the special group had joined a club and had a holiday during the preceding year and the old people in the special group rated significantly higher in scores for general activities than the clients in the comparison group.

5. *'More clients in the special than in the comparison group will show improvement in their attitudes to their present situation as measured by the attitude score.'*

This hypothesis was upheld. We have shown that the clients in the special group had improved significantly in their 'morale' and in their attitudes to the outside world, while the old people in the comparison group improved very little in these respects.

6. *'At the end of the social work period clients in the special group will have fewer social needs than clients in the comparison group and the decrease in needs will be greater in the special than in the comparison group.'*

This hypothesis was upheld in both respects.

7. *'Clients who were initially severely emotionally disturbed or had seriously disturbed interpersonal relationships will show greater improvement in the special than in the comparison group.'*

Although numbers were too small to test this hypothesis rigorously the indications are that clients in the special group who were severely disturbed and had seriously disturbed interpersonal relationships improved more as measured by their scores on the morale factor than similar clients in the comparison group.

Consumer Reactions

The clients' own perceptions and evaluations of the help they had received from social workers during the experimental period revealed significant differences between the groups. The old people's reports on the regularity of visits, which had taken place at least monthly, corresponded reasonably well with recorded visits of the social workers in the special group. A significantly higher proportion of clients in the special group felt that the social workers' visits had been of help to them. These clients' spontaneous comments showed more warmth towards their social workers and greater perception of their personalities and more awareness of the supportive and caring nature of their relationships with them. Clients in both groups mentioned a great variety of practical help they had valued; holidays and clubs, aids and appliances, and domiciliary services heading the list. Clients in the special group mentioned almost three times as many helpful practical services performed by the social workers as the clients in the comparison group.

Seven per cent of the clients in the special and 15 per cent in the comparison group found the visits of no help. In some instances the help had not been relevant to the need as perceived by the client, some clients had very disturbed personalities for whom nothing was right, a few refused services altogether from a fierce and unreasonable sense of independence and some did not really need any help. Although the clients in the special group felt more satisfied and mentioned more concrete help provided by their social workers yet when asked what else ought to be done, more of them made suggestions than among the comparison group – money and housing topping the list. Perhaps their recent experience taught them that there was no need to 'put up with things'; they felt confident enough to raise their expectations with a resulting decrease in apathy.

In general these results make sense. One would not expect *individual* social work effort to impinge on broad social conditions, such as housing or income, nor would one expect any improvement in general health in this very aged group, though one might have hoped for some relief of minor discomforts. On the other hand one did hope that social work would result in a reduction of practical needs and in an improvement in social and psychological functioning. The less trained social workers of the welfare department achieved a good deal, though not as much as their trained colleagues in alleviating their clients' practical needs. The trained workers also brought about some improvement in their clients' activities and in their feelings and attitudes, and these assessments find confirmation in the clients' own reactions and comments about the help they had received.

Size of Caseload and Outcome

Readers may doubt whether these results throw any light on the relative effectiveness of social work carried out by professionally trained social workers and by experienced welfare officers who did not have professional social work training. Critics may argue: granted that a number of statistically significant differences and many smaller differences emerged in outcome favouring the special group, does this not merely indicate that the special group responded to more intensive attention? Is it not likely that the differences found are due to differences in caseloads and pressures of work rather than to the quality of work done? There are many indications that size of caseload affected the results reported. On practically every count – number of contacts with clients in the project, contacts with agencies, and number of items of practical help provided, the average input of the project workers was twice that of their colleagues in the welfare department.

Strong suggestions are emerging from other studies (Reid and Shyne, op. cit.) that intensive and focused effort, particularly within the first two months of a case, is more effective than open-ended long-drawn-out social work. Similar trends were noticeable in our study. The project social workers' first twenty cases which had a great deal of attention during the first two months after referral improved considerably more than cases taken on during the middle period when these workers were carrying their maximum caseload and could not grapple with their clients' problems in this immediate and intensive manner. In the comparison group, where effort was more evenly distributed throughout the study period, the rate of improvement among the first, middle and last twenty cases followed no particular pattern. However, size of caseload was not the only factor determining size and nature of input. For instance, we observed that the project workers expended much more effort on their small caseload at the beginning of the study than on their equally small caseloads towards the end of the experiment, and we concluded that the workers' motivation may have played a part. We also discovered that the number of visits and the amount of practical help given were significantly associated with reduction in practical needs, but much less with improvement in psychological functioning. In short, the amount of input which is almost certainly related to size of caseload, is associated with improvement in the practical situation. More complex factors, possibly related to the quality of the casework and to the client-worker relationship, the personality of the client and his life situation seem to account for improvement in functioning, attitudes and feelings. Comments clients made about their social workers and the nature of their contact with them strengthen these hunches.

There are other indications that the differences in outcome are not merely a reflection of the social worker's availability and the amount of input but also reflect differences in the helper's perceptions and techniques of working. For example, the project social workers diagnosed more problems and hence found more to tackle, and this applied particularly to less obvious difficulties in social and emotional functioning. This fuller social diagnosis engendered more varied ways of working: the project social workers encouraged more expression of feelings and discussion of interpersonal relationships and they combined provision of services with casework and work with relatives more often than did the workers in the comparison group. We also found that the project social workers' input varied sharply with their clients' needs; they worked selectively, putting in twice as much effort with those clients whose need was judged to be 'considerable' by the independent assessors as they did with those whose need for social work was judged to be slight. The social workers in the comparison group did not work as selectively as their more trained colleagues.

There is a further interesting difference in 'set' which may have influenced outcome; the project social workers knew that they had at most 10 months to make any difference to their clients' lives. The case discussions with the project director may also have made a contribution in keeping goals firmly in mind. Three questions were invariably asked: what were the problems to begin with, what had been done and what were the plans for future action or treatment? The social workers in the comparison group had no particular time target, nor did they have similar opportunities for reassessing their cases and reformulating goals.

As far as this study is concerned we draw the tentative conclusion that while size of caseload was an important factor in determining certain aspects of outcome it was not by itself sufficient to explain all the differences that occurred. There is evidence that motivation, skill and a goal-directed approach also played a part in determining outcome.

It is clear that future experiments should seek to control workload and caseload factors if at all possible. Such studies could be designed in two ways. If relative effects of different treatment are to be investigated then it would be desirable to keep the caseloads in the control and experimental groups as similar as possible. If on the other hand it is the intention to explore the effect of size of caseload on outcome then one would seek to vary the size of caseload experimentally, while keeping the type of treatment essentially the same for both groups.

Training as a Contributory Factor in Outcome
Another question which this study cannot answer in any definitive way is how much training contributed to outcome. Since only two trained workers dealt with the experimental group it is reasonable to suggest that it was their personalities, natural gifts, their enhanced motivation resulting from this assignment for which they were selected, and the opportunities for regular team discussions which gave them the advantage over their colleagues. Once more it seems impossible, with the evidence available, to disentangle all these influences without more detailed study. It is our impression that differences in outcome were not merely due to clients receiving more attention from two highly motivated and gifted social workers, but that their similar casework training did contribute substantially to their ability to assess the clients' social situation and their needs in a comprehensive way. Their training may have enabled them to formulate a rounded social work plan which combined the use of many community resources with casework. Training probably sensitized them to the less obvious problems and helped them to work differentially, according to people's needs. At the same time there is little doubt that the workers' experience and personal gifts, the spur of the unusual time-limited experiment, and the opportunities presented by regular and stimulating case discussions also played a part.

Consumer Aspects

We saw in the chapter on consumer aspects that general questions such as 'Do you feel you have had enough help over the last year?' brought forth undifferentiated and stereotyped replies. More specific inquiries about the visits from social workers and the help derived from them brought out rich and highly individualized comments, as did a question asking for the old people's opinions of what else could or ought to be done to help them. Even very old people with generally low expectations, if encouraged to comment, can express opinions about what they want. Much more needs to be learnt about how clients perceive their most pressing needs, how they see social workers and what they consider to be effective social work. For instance, among this small sample of elderly welfare clients it seemed quite clear that the old people rejected a rather impersonal services-orientated approach, as well as a very personal one which did not heed their practical needs. Their comments also showed how important a consistent willingness to help in any situation was to them and how much security they derived from knowing exactly where to turn in time of need, confident that a response would be forthcoming.

Implications for Other Services

In this small experiment some of the more generally acknowledged difficulties in helping the aged stood out clearly. One-fifth of the clients in both groups were still in very unsuitable housing at the end of the experiment. It is now gradually realized that the very old, who have lived for the most part of their lives in one small neighbourhood, are most successfully rehoused within the familiar streets to which they have grown attached and which constitute their world imbued with many memories. The less an old person is able to experience other environments by going out, the more he clings to the one he knows. A move, even ten minutes away, can mean the end of his accustomed way of life; for example, the life-line services of a neighbour may be disrupted which can be more vital than the occasional visits from children. Thus offers of rehousing were refused on several occasions because it meant a move away from a familiar neighbourhood. An alternative solution, the refurbishing or readaptation of old and inconvenient premises often did not seem feasible because the property was scheduled to be pulled down in two or three years' time. Yet for the clients it meant spending the last years of their lives, when increasing infirmity calls for more comfort, in most inconvenient housing. In this way ambitious and benevolent long-term housing policies clashed with the urgent needs of individuals who would never live to see the splendid shape of things to come.

Few clients, some 3 per cent, went into residential accommodation during the ten months of the field experiment; and at the end of the experiment only a further 3 per cent of these incapacitated and very aged clients were on the waiting list for residential accommodation. This may reflect the old people's great unwillingness to give up their independence but it is also an eloquent commentary on the amount of community care and support the borough provides for their elderly citizens. However, while few of the old people needed total care, the assessors considered that some 10 per cent required the partial care of warden-supervised housing. This type of provision hardly existed in the area. Hence a number of physically or mentally infirm clients lived a precarious existence on their own, a source of anxiety to themselves, their neighbours and more distant relatives. Another difficulty related to housing which caused some frustration to both clients and helpers was adaptations within the home, designed to make life easier and safer for the old person, such as grab rails, ramps, etc. Even this progressive authority did not employ any experts to advise on adaptations or to carry out measurements. This meant that social workers who had no particular training or expertise in this field had to make suggestions and take measurements. Their suggestions may not have always been appropriate and their measurements, on occasions, proved inaccurate. In addition, delays usually due to administrative hold-ups caused hardship in some cases.

Here we touch on larger issues of rigidities and lack of urgency in bureaucratic structures which militate against decisions nearer the field level.

Another administrative problem affecting the delivery of services was transport to clubs. The spread of clubs and day centres and the relatively high participation rate is a particularly encouraging feature of the community services for the handicapped and elderly in this borough. Unfortunately, the transport arrangements severely limited the use that could be made of these facilities. It seems important to bear in mind the interrelationships of the various parts of the welfare services. A great expansion of one part – additional social workers or clubs – may be less beneficial in the long run than a more modest, but balanced, expansion of all interrelated parts of a service which would put its resources to optimal use.

One of the most interesting challenges encountered in this experiment was collaboration with volunteers. We have described the difficulties of keeping young volunteers interested and of locating suitable older voluntary visitors; and we have referred to the considerable amount of regular help neighbours gave on a purely informal basis. At the end of the experiment the assessors considered that only a small proportion of clients – between 6 per cent and 7 per cent – still required a voluntary visitor. The caseworkers on the other hand felt that the rather restricted lives of many of their clients could have been enriched by volunteers from the neighbourhood; they could have taken them out, rendered little services such as sewing, shopping, giving them a hairdo, cooking the odd meal or just sitting chatting. As mentioned before, volunteer school-children could only be available late in the afternoon when the old people were often tired; and the young people at times did not see the point of 'just visiting'. The old people for their part occasionally felt that they gained little understanding and companionship from the very young. However, there were notable exceptions, when for example the old client would eagerly look forward to the next instalment in a boy/girl romance. It proved difficult to match individual client and volunteer, partly because the volunteer was allocated by special liaison officers employed by the welfare department and the social workers had little choice in the matter. The young people received little if any help to prepare and train them for their voluntary tasks. As they worked mainly under the guidance of their teachers and the liaison officers, the contacts between the volunteers and the social worker on the case were very loose and ill defined. Yet the social workers wished to be in closer touch with the volunteers and to guide them a little in their work. Ideally, it seemed to us, each social worker should have worked with a group of volunteers assigned to his cases, meeting them regularly to discuss their activities. It also seemed to us that a fresh and imaginative drive was indicated in some districts of the borough in order to find older volunteers from the neighbourhood itself. House to house surveys or well-advertised local campaigns might have brought some response. In one district a house-to-house survey, conducted by one of the volunteer services liaison officers produced several very suitable visitors for the elderly.

We drew the tentative conclusion from our limited experience, that more systematic thinking needed to be done about recruitment and preparation of volunteers for the elderly, as well as about roles and functions of organizers of volunteers, sponsors of volunteers such as teachers, and the social workers in charge of the cases. The relationships between these different partners in the enterprise also needed to be more clearly defined. Meanwhile the Aves Report has produced some helpful guidelines. (Aves, G. M., Chairman, 1969.)

Another aspect of the project which provided much food for thought was the collaboration between the social services, the clients' doctors and the health services generally. We noted the reluctance of some general practitioners to intervene actively with the very old and we discovered how little general practitioners knew about the mental condition of their patients. We also observed that the minor miseries of old age, such as foot discomforts, poor sight and hearing, giddiness, urinary symptoms, constipation and poor sleep had increased in both groups, despite the attention the clients had received from the social services. It became clear that the social workers had not been able to spot most of these minor disabilities nor had they been brought to the notice of the doctors by the clients themselves.

How could these clients be helped more adequately? Closer teamwork between social worker and doctor seems essential. This might be achieved by part-time attachments of social workers to general practice or by regular consultations and reviews of old clients on the general practitioners' list. It also seems desirable to bring in the community nurse for regular screening functions. At the time of writing several studies are in progress which attempt to work out simple geriatric screening procedures which could be carried out by non-medical personnel[1] (Williamsons et al. 1966). Such screening tests would probably have to take place in the homes of those over eighty, as these patients often seemed resigned to disabilities and discomforts which can be relieved. It has also occurred to us that the advice of geriatricians should be available to the social service department concerned with the community care of the elderly rather like that of psychiatrists who are attached to health departments, in order to give

[1] Dr J. M. G. Wilson and his colleagues at the London School of Hygiene and Tropical Medicine are carrying out a study to validate screening tests which can be administered by nurses to old people in their own homes in order to detect medical and social needs, and to show that the disabilities uncovered by such tests can frequently be alleviated.

consultative help to social workers dealing with mentally ill and handicapped clients.

Implications for the Social Work Task

This study and experience generally suggest that the social worker's task can be as varied in the field of old age as in any other age group. Social work with these old clients had certain characteristic features which may have relevance to social work with the aged generally.

Environmental and practical support of all kinds probably assumes greater importance in this age group than in any other, particularly for those living alone or with slender family resources.

Since old people coming to the notice of welfare departments are often frail and physically or mentally handicapped, more determined efforts at reaching out and holding on to clients may have to be made than with younger, more independent people.

As with the very young, this reaching out may entail protecting clients from the neglect and apathy of others, or from their own neglect. In these situations the principle of self-determination is of limited validity; yet it is difficult to delineate the degree of responsibility social workers should be prepared to assume on behalf of their very old and dependent clients.

The social worker's role as an enabler, making needs explicit and helping clients to accept services which they need and to which they are entitled was an important one among old people whose expectations were often low, for whom the concept of welfare was still reminiscent of the Poor Law and whose Victorian ethics of independence were still noticeable.

This enabling role on occasions becomes an advocacy role, helping an old person to get to know and obtain his rights.

Collaboration with a host of other statutory and voluntary agencies on behalf of the elderly client, acting as a co-ordinator of these services, ensuring that they function smoothly and appropriately, emerged as a central task in the present fragmented personal social services for the aged. New and challenging problems await the attention of social workers, such as the development of a more helpful partnership with volunteers, or experimentation with more flexible roles for home helps.

The importance and validity of a careful and sound initial assessment was strikingly demonstrated. Among this group of welfare clients who ranged from ordinary old people with few practical needs to severely incapacitated clients with complex problems, it was possible to assess broadly, in one interview, the degree and nature of social work need. This suggests that initial assessments should wherever possible be carried out, or at least be closely supervised by senior and experienced social workers so that resources can be allocated appropriately.

Clients in the older age range whose infirmities, physical or mental, create problems for themselves or their environment can make as taxing demands on the skills of trained social workers as any other group of clients. We learnt during the course of the project that casework with the elderly demanded certain special skills, adaptations and restraints on the part of the social workers. These included awareness of the old people's slower pace, of the accumulation of loss and depression, of the growing restrictions in life space and the increasing difficulty in absorbing new experiences or change. Casework was less concerned with modifying maladaptive behaviour or bringing about different perceptions of the world or changes in attitudes. Instead of change from within, social work had to contrive to find small environmental supports or compensatory experiences such as clubs, work groups, a holiday and so on. Thus, casework interviews would not delve into past conflicts which may have been at the root of present difficulties, but they would gently clarify as much of the present problems and the personal situation as was necessary in order to bring the right kind of support to bear. Expression of feelings about painful situations often turned into reassuring and emotionally satisfying reminiscences which can help the old person to regain a sense of positive worth and identity. We noticed that in working with the old the case worker is more likely to slip into the role of a substitute son or daughter or grandchild. It seemed important to beware of this and to seek for more long-term substitutes such as volunteers, friends at clubs, or neighbours, since the casework relationship can only rarely, if ever, become a substitute for an enduring friendship.

As already indicated, the identification of minor physical disabilities and discomforts and ensuring that they receive attention emerged as an important caring function, which is often overlooked. Whether this should become part of the social worker's task in close collaboration with the general practitioner or should also include a community nurse, is an open question needing further study.

In this small experiment it proved possible for a social worker to identify those old people who appeared to have an insufficient diet and social workers were able to exert some influence on diet as part of their social work effort.

In our judgement about a third of this mixed sample of welfare clients did not need the help of a trained social worker. Such clients had one or more of the following attributes: their disabilities did not seriously impede functioning, their morale was good and they were well supported by family, friends or the social services. These clients, we thought, could benefit from occasional review visits by in-service-trained welfare assistants working under the supervision of a trained social worker.

Implications for Training of Social Workers

Although our experience was limited it was probably not atypical, and since social work with the elderly is expanding, implications for social work training are important.

If social workers are to develop more than an informed layman's understanding of the ageing process and its physical, psychological and sociological concomitants, more attention and expertise will have to be devoted to this subject in the teaching of human development, social behaviour and social structure and in field training. In the teaching of social work methods, the part social work can play in the care of the elderly is much neglected. Yet it provides singularly rich material for the comparative study of different social work methods; principles and practice of residential care are virtually unexplored in this field; group work of various kinds in clubs and day centres is growing, but needs much further stimulation and study; advocacy and social action on behalf of this unvocal group are appropriate in certain circumstances; community work has great potentialities, for example, recruitment of neighbourhood-based volunteers, encouragement of self-help – the 'young olds' helping the 'old olds' – development of local social networks for isolated old people; social planning in relation to the known physical, social and psychological needs of the elderly and their more positive integration into the local community and society generally and not merely into 'the community of the old' is also a field worthy of study; and last but not least there is casework with its distinctive characteristics in relation to this age group.

The Way Ahead

Finally, we wish to return to the criticisms voiced about social work experiments and to examine shortly how our field experiment has stood up to them. These criticisms referred to the client's motivation when he was randomly assigned to a kind of treatment he had not sought, to the vague objectives pursued by social work; they questioned how relevant to the client's problems the methods of social work had been, and they raised the issue of long-term effects which may escape measurement. Our field experiment we feel, was sufficiently rooted in the ordinary fieldwork situation not to arouse puzzled suspicion; its objectives were deliberately operational and modest in scope and in keeping with the limited adjustment one could reasonably expect in this age group; a determined, if crude attempt was made to describe and measure the social work input, and by adopting a 'multi-level' approach we tried to make social work relevant to the wide ranging needs of old people; since death was round the corner for many of the clients, the possible long-term effects were not so important.

This final evaluation is not meant to convey smug satisfaction with the modest results achieved. Many questions are left unanswered or partially answered, not least of which is what type and level of training is necessary for different kinds of social work tasks. Nor do we wish to paper over the gaps in methodology, notably our comparative failure to identify more precisely the psychological and inter-actional components in the case work process which may have influenced outcome in relation to functioning, attitudes and feelings. Nor are we happy about the gaps revealed in social work, especially our relative inability to spot and ensure treatment of the miseries of old age.

What we do wish to convey is our belief that if social workers were prepared to define their middle-range goals in more precise operational terms, to describe and where appropriate to categorize and measure their social work activities, to tolerate independent assessments and to heed their clients' evaluations, then we could take a great leap ahead in any sphere of social work we cared to study. We could gradually get closer to determining the relative effectiveness of different types of intervention in different situations. Training and deployment of limited resources could then be based, at least partially, on tested evidence rather than on commitment to certain methods of social work. And this, we think, is true service to our clients.

References
Aves, G. M., Chairman (1969): *The Voluntary Worker in the Social Services,* Allen and Unwin.
Williamson, J., Lowther, C. P. and Gray, S. (1966): 'The Use of Health Visitors in Preventive Geriatrics', *Geront. Clin.* No. 8, p. 362.

APPENDIX I

TABLE 1

HOUSEHOLD TENURE
(By persons in private households)

Welfare Clients compared with Borough Population
(Percentage distribution)

Tenure	Welfare clients (N=294*)	Borough population (N=279,560)
Owner occupied	7	14
Rented: from L.A.	43	44
privately furnished	3	4
privately unfurnished	47	38
Totals	100	100

Source: 1966 Sample Census for Greater London, Table 9.

* No evidence for 6 people.

TABLE 2

HOUSEHOLD AMENITIES
Welfare Clients compared with Borough Population
(Percentage distribution)

Use	Household Amenities					
	Hot-water tap		Fixed bath		Indoor W.C.	
	Welfare clients (N=294‡)	Borough population (N=100,860)	Welfare clients (N=294‡)	Borough population (N=100,860)	Welfare clients (N=293†)	Borough population (N=100,580)
Sole use	63	66	48	55	61	65
Shared	1	5	4	11	11	13
None	36	29	48	34	28*	22**
Totals	100	100	100	100	100	100

Source: 1966 Sample Census County Report for Greater London, Table 12.

* All the old people who had no indoor W.C. had the use of an outdoor W.C

** All but 0·36 of the population had use of an outdoor W.C.

† No Evidence for 7 people.

‡ No Evidence for 6 people.

TABLE 3

CLASSIFICATION BY DIAGNOSTIC GROUPINGS OF 68 WELFARE CLIENTS
IN SEVERELY ILL CATEGORY*

Diagnostic group		No. of welfare clients
Cardio-respiratory		19
Cerebral		26
i) organic brain syndrome	12	
ii) other evidence of cerebral arterial disease, e.g. Parkinsonism; stroke.	14	
Malignancy		7
Multiple disease groups		12
Other (e.g. diabetes; myxoedema)		4
Total		68

* The prognostic classification of severity was based on the *main* condition present. A subject suffering from advanced malignant disease might, incidentally, be suffering from heart disease.

TABLE 4

COMPARISON OF REPORTED PREVALENCE OF SOME DISABILITIES AMONG 283 SOUTH LONDON WELFARE CLIENTS AGED 70+
WITH STUDIES OF OTHER AGED POPULATIONS
(Percentage distributions)

Year and area of survey	Character of sample	No. in sample	Sex distrib.	Age group	Chiropodial problems	Loss of Bladder control	Giddiness	Difficulty in seeing	Deafness
1966–1968 South London borough	Consecutive series of selected welfare clients	283	M= 73 F = 210	70+	68	48	43	28	31
1962–1963 Edinburgh	Random sample of patients aged 65+ of three general practices	200	M= 91 F = 109	65+	47	18	—	36	36
1962 National	2 random samples of persons aged 65+	4,209	M=1674 F=2535	65+	30	—	—	31*	33*
1961 Lewisham	Random sample of local residents	1,287	M= 536 F = 751	65+	59	—	—	—	30

1961 Swansea	Random sample of persons aged 65+	228	M = 99 F = 129	65+	—	—	50	—	—
	All residents aged 80+ traceable in records of: a) General practitioner's b) Local authority Health & Welfare Department c) Hospitals & nursing homes also: d) Respondents to advertisements e) Names recommended to interviewer in the course of the survey								
1956 – 1957 Stockport		2,072	M = 656 F = 1416	80+	—	24	—	—	—
1945 – 1947 Wolverhampton	Random sample of women aged 60+ and men aged 65+	477	M = 143 F = 334	65+ 60+	—	—	52	—	31

— No evidence on these items.

* Only based on questions asked in the second stage of the survey (i.e., to 1,567 persons).

205

TABLE 5

PSYCHIATRIC DISORDERS OF 46 WELFARE CLIENTS

Disorder		Number of clients
Organic brain syndrome		30
Functional disorders		16
Anxiety neurosis	5	
Schizophrenia & paranoid psychosis	5	
Affective disorder	3	
Alcoholism	2	
Personality disorder	1	
Total		46

TABLE 6

COMPARATIVE MOVEMENT FROM FIRST ASSESSMENT TO SECOND ASSESSMENT

Item	Special group (N=110)	Comparison group (N=104)	Probability Level
Belonging to a club			
Joined a club	16	0	} p 0·01
Did not join	66	73	
Already a club member	28	30	
No evidence	0	1	
Holiday within the last year			
Last year but not previous year	20	2	} p 0·01
No holiday last year	61	66	
Holiday in both years	29	33	
No evidence	0	3	
Satisfaction			
No longer dissatisfied	14	3	} p ·01
Still dissatisfied	7	13	
Not dissatisfied originally	84	85	
No evidence	5	3	
Depression			
Reduced to 'Normal'	21	7	} p ·01
Not reduced to 'Normal'	53	59	
Originally 'Normal'	24	27	
No evidence	3	3	
Reduction in personal problems			
Reduced number of pronounced or moderate problems	25	12	} p ·05
Not reduced	39	47	
Slight or no problems initially	46	45	
Deterioration in medical condition	(N=101)	(N=96)	
Deteriorated to 'Seriously Ill' category	4	15	} p 0·01
Did not deteriorate to 'Seriously Ill' category	80	68	
Already 'Seriously Ill'	17	13	

APPENDIX 2

METHODS OF ANALYSIS

Owing to the great amount of data from the social and medical questionnaires (unsuitable for machine analysis in their present form), it was decided to compile work sheets – these were used for making comparisons for all questions between answers given by the two groups and on the two occasions. The work sheets had the added advantage that they could be used as working documents by all members of the research team working on the project.

At the end of the field work, a list of survivors (those who had had two full assessments) was compiled, also lists of those who died during the survey, were permanently in hospital and who had entered residential accommodation. In addition, five questionnaires were discarded for the comparison, on the grounds that only meagre information had been obtained at one or both assessments.

Talks were then held with the Research Director to decide which key items were suitable for the correlation matrix. Evidence from other research has shown the desirability of keeping matrices for analysis to a reasonable size, in particular with respect to the interpretation of 'factors' emerging. Although it might appear that this selection of items was somewhat arbitrary, in fact this was less than apparent. The questionnaire had been originally designed for two purposes: to describe the social and medical conditions of old people and to assess changes due to different types of social work. Some questions were relevant to both purposes, but many, clearly, only referred to the former.

Items were chosen to achieve adequate coverage of those areas for which beneficial results arising from good social work might be expected: for example whereas the decorations of the home and attitudes of the elderly to housing might improve, the type of accommodation and amenities, such as baths and toilets etc., would probably be the same after a period of ten months. It was also necessary to exclude sub-questions inapplicable to certain respondents, e.g. the hours worked by the home help, or 'who cooked hot meals for those unable to manage the cooking for themselves'. Selection of items from the medical questionnaire was more difficult, but in general we chose those items which summarized the data in some appropriate area, *viz*. general state of health, breathlessness, mobility and function, depression, confusion. Finally, it was desirable not to mix categorized data resulting from a 'Yes/No' type answer, with answers presented in some form of rating scale – in fact the latter type was more prevalent and all the selected items could be quantified in this way.

Transfer forms were then designed to cover the selected items. A novel method was used to minimize the number of bi-polar factors. Each item was coded in the same direction with respect to its rating scale, i.e. the best/most favourable items were coded (and subsequently punched) as code No. 1, whereas the unfavourable/detrimental ratings were all coded as 3, 4 or 5. Coding was carried out question by question direct from the work sheets, but a 100 per cent. check was made, case by case, from the original questionnaires. Another innovation was used for coding instructions to avoid errors arising from misreading. Instead of the usual briefing notes, the coding instructions for each item were typed on to separate cards, and all cards collected in order using split rings. Thus a coder coding say question 6, would have the coding instructions for *that question alone* propped up in front of her. Transfer forms were prepared for both the first and second assessments, for each survivor.

The codes for the first assessments were then punched on to Holerith cards and tables of distributions (and percentages) examined. One item with poor discriminative power was excluded at this stage. The cards were then transferred to IBM-1131-03C computer, and product-moment intercorrelations calculated; these were then submitted to a principal components programme, and analysis into 7–11 (inclusive) 'factors' carried out, using both Varimax and Promax rotations. After examination of the computer sheets, we accepted the 11 'factor' solution with Varimax (orthogonal) loadings.* These 11 factors accounted for 60·1 per cent. of the variance. In view of heterogeneity of the data and the high error variance expected from this population, it was decided to consider only loadings of 0·40 and above. This gave clean factors', using all but five of the 48 items. These factor loadings are appended.

Factor scores were then calculated. If an old person had the lowest scale rating, he received the maximum score for that item; if he had a high (satisfactory) rating, he received zero, and if his rating was somewhere between these two, his score was adjusted proportionately. Scores for each factor for each person were obtained by summing the relevant item scores and normalizing for the number of items included. These factor scores were calculated for the two groups separately, and for the first and second assessments of each group. Means and variances were obtained, and a check made using the variance ratio test to ensure homogeneity of variance. (Fortunately the

---

* The Varimax and Promax loadings were virtually identical, but the Varimax had the benefit of orthogonality.

numbers in the two groups were similar, *viz.* 104 and 110). The differences between the group means were tested using the t test.

FACTORS

Loadings

Factor 1 'Capacity and Mobility' (var.=10·67)
0·89 Personal incapacity score
0·85 Functional mobility
0·74 Activity score
0·77 Effective mobility level for most difficult task
0·76 Functional movement
0·73 Household incapacity score
0·73 Ability to manage stairs

Factor 2 'Depression' (var.=9·61)
0·90 How long does the depression last?
0·90 How often do you feel depressed?
0·89 Do you get depressed nowadays?
0·74 Do you ever feel like crying?
0·61 What do you feel life holds for you?
0·48 How do you find the time passes?

Factor 3 'Morale' (var.=6·12)
0·69 Social attitudes to outside world
0·63 Satisfaction with life at the moment
0·59 Worries
0·63 Assessment of personal problems
0·54 Loneliness

Factor 4 'Practical Needs' (var.=5·80)
0·82 Number of practical social service needs
0·78 Total number of practical needs
0·65 Indications for social work

Factor 5 'Confusion' (var.=4·67)
0·80 Medical assessor's classification of confusion
0·80 Tooting Bec score
0·54 Medical assessor's classification of physical health and prognosis

Factor 6 'Physical Environment' (var.=4·34)
0·76 Suitability of housing
0·67 Condition of decorations
0·51 Assessment of environmental difficulties

Loadings

Factors continued

0·47 Condition of furnishings
0·44 Satisfaction with housing

Factor 7 'Finance' (var. = 4·08)
0·69 Sufficiency of income
0·61 Difficulty in meeting expenses
0·48 Social class

Factor 8 'Social Isolation' (var. = 4·07)
0·64 Assessment of social isolation
0·63 Number of people seen yesterday
0·56 Age of client

Factor 9 'Social Services' (var. = 4·01)
0·85 Number of subsidiary services received
0·83 Frequency of having had a holiday

Factor 10 'General Health' (var. = 3·51)
0·57 Breathlessness
0·51 Old person's opinion of health

Factor 11* 'Diet' (var. = 3·22)
0·71 Client lives alone
—0·64 Diet score

* Factor very dubious.

INDEX

Abel-Smith, B. 52
A comparison of the average weekly consumption or purchase of milk, cheese, bread and eggs among three samples of old people (Table III. 11) 67
Additional help desired by welfare clients (Table VIII. 3) 182
Additional help needed by welfare clients as judged by social work assessors (Table III. 15b) 75
Age-sex distribution of 41 local authority social workers carrying 104 cases in comparison group (Table V. 2) 101
alcoholics 72, 163
anaemia in old people 63
assessment techniques used to select clients 35–40; importance of 197–9
assessors 37, 73, 85, 88, 126, 130; medical 39, 51, 68, 76, 98, 106, 137, 138, 157, 160, 161, 162, 163, 164, 166, 168, 169, 186; social 37, 57, 74, 76, 107, 145, 171, 186
Assessors' clinical judgements (Table VI. 8) 149
Assessors' judgements of presence of practical needs (Table VI. 7) 146
Average number of visits, contacts with other agencies and items of practical help, compared with the assessors' judgements of 'indications for social work' (Table V. 11) 126
Average weekly income of 238 welfare clients willing to give this information (Table III. 8) 56
Aves, G. M. 196
Aves Report 196

behaviour therapists 25

Benjamin Rose Institute, study carried out in 28
Blenkner, M. 27, 28, 105
blindness in old people 65
Booth, C. 56
Briar, Scott 22
British Association of Social Workers 21
Brown, Gordon E. 28, 105
Butrym, Zofia 22

capacity, and attitudes 60–2; and health of old people 136–9
Capacity and health (Table VI. 2) 136
case histories, detailed 72, 157–66
caseload, size of and outcome 112–13, 190–2
Caseloads of social workers in special and comparison groups in the four areas of the borough (Table V. 1) 99
cases, assessing progress of individual 152–6
casework service 28, 76–7
clubs and day centres attended by the aged 40, 48, 62, 72, 76, 79, 85, 114, 116, 129, 159, 162, 164, 166, 177, 189, 194
Cole, D. 56
Community Service Society of New York 27, 28, 31, 105
'comparison' group 33, 41, 42, 98, 99, 103, 126; compared to 'special' group 83–97, 130–3, 134, 137–8, 142, 147; deterioration of morale in 164–6; differences in outcome between special group and 150–1; improvement of morale in 160–2; outcome and reactions to work carried out in 187–8
computer, use of in this study 152, 209